Muscular Integrated In-depth Therapy

Marijane Lescroart

Muscular Integrated In-depth Therapy

Marijane Lescroart

Published by:
Marijane Lescroart
2414 Pinercrest Dr.
Santa Rosa, CA, USA

A CIP record for this book is available from the Library of Congress Cataloging-in-Publication Data

ISBN: 9798335763400

Printed in USA

Acknowledgements

I would like to thank my dear friend Giselle Reese, who left this dimension in July 2003. Without her guidance and direction, my therapy would not have been applied to paper.

I would also like to thank Gerry and Georgia Tripp for their encouragement and research. Their help gave me many hours to grow and shape my work.

Thank you to all my teachers: Alice Smith, Pam Grant, Paul Dennission, Carla Henniford, Joanne Shaw, Ric Levendosky, and Sue Metzger. You gave me the challenges, motivation, hope, support and courage to step from the past to the future with strength, ease and peace. Each of you add your own little touch to my work.

In honor of your time, insight & support, I give this Integration In-depth therapy to the world.

Contents

The doctor of the future will give no medicine but will interest his patients in the care of the human frame, in diet, and in the cause and prevention of disease.

-Thomas Edison

CHAPTER I

Introduction to Integrated Therapy

What is Integrated Therapy?

Integrated In-Depth Therapy is a technique that I developed in order to heal my own life. It wasn't deliberate. In fact, it came about more by happenstance. It was the cumulative result of years and years of study and research--taking a variety of classes and reading everything that I could get my hands on to help my individual situation. As I tell my own story, you will see how, I learned to use

Integrated therapy in my own life. And I found
that I could better deal with my polio, with
food allergies, and with a variety of other
things the more I used it. I also learned to
communicate better, eliminate seizures and
other physical and emotional issues that
hindered me having a normal life. Through
Integrated therapy, I even began to see some
improvements in my son who suffers from his
own disablities. After several years of success
in healing myself and improving the conditions
my son had, I felt that I had something to offer
to others. The ability to help others has been
the ultimate test of this technique. And now,
through this book, it is my desire to teach
others how to heal as well--To heal naturally,
through this Integrated In-Depth therapy
technique and to heal without the use of
pharmeceuticals.

In my own health journey as a young
child, I was blessed to experience initial
closeness with my twin brother. It is a bond
that very few people get to experience. At six
weeks gestation, my mother contracted
Bulbar's paralysis Polio and suddenly, my
brother Eric and I's peaceful world in the
womb was thrown into a shock. I was to
witness his dramatic passing and the grief and
shock of that loss sent me into a coma that I
didn't wake from until I was born at twenty
four weeks...I was just over two pounds and 13
inches long.

Being born so small, I spent the first few
months of my life in the hospital. My parents
and my four siblings would come to visit every
day while I was in the hospital. It was
honestly all a trauma, and as a result, I had

seizures and was on a lung ventilator from the time that I was born until they felt that I was strong enough to go home. Later in life, it was the long lasting effects of my traumatic birth that would have me searching for answers.

When I decided to invent this technique, it was kind of by accident--a cumulation of all of my research and putting things together one by one--and Muscular Integrated Therapy (MIIT) was born. In 1991 I began learning how to do Brain Gym from a woman named Susan Metzger in Guerneville, CA. I took a couple of Brain Gym classes and I actually really enjoyed them. She told me there was a technique that I might like and we began working to set some goals for my health. I agreed, and we started some communication balancing. (AKA, The Brain Gym techique). I was extremely interested and it all seemed like it was the kind of thing that was right up my alley. I started learning Brain Gym 101 for communication, and our first goal was for me to be able to communicate efficiently. This was a huge goal for me, because the paralysis from the Polio made it difficult to speak.

I faced several challenges while I was going through the Brain Gym program. I was frequently dehydrated alot of the time. And I must have drank at least seven or eight gallons of water during the balance program. I was also going through a divorce from my husband around that time, which added to the challenge as I was trying to tackle my health. That first goal was quite a big deal to me because I wanted to work on trying to get my driver's license. At that time my communication skills were very limited and I still required a lot of

water during treatments. But once I started
noticing real changes, I got more and more
excited about the prospect of my health
changing for the better. I knew right away
that it was going to be an interesting tool.

After a period of time, I started speaking
a lot more. Before those treatments, I didn't
speak very much at all, and I tended to be more
of an observer sitting around watching
everything going on around me rather than
interacting and getting involved in things. As I
started to improve, my Brain Gym instructor
gave me more and more tools and I went back
to her for a few more sessions. It was then
that she told me that she was going to be
teaching a Brain Gym class and she asked if I
would be interested in joining them. She
thought that it could really help me. So I
pinched and scraped my pennies together and I
went to her first class. It was a very good class
and I finished Brain Gym 101 Balance. But she
planned on teaching more. She said that she
would be doing what was called a Vision Circle,
so after that, I took a 24 hour class called
Vision 101. Then I continued on to do Vision
Circles, which was yet another 24-hour class.
The Brain Gym program requires that you take
every class twice before you get teacher
practicum. So the next weekend I did another
24-hour class for Vision Circles. This was at
the very beginning of Brain Gym, so I started
to take the classes and even traveled to Arizona
and Los Angeles to take other ones. In fact,
almost every weekend I was taking another
Brain Gym class and moving further into the
program. By the end of 1994 I had completed
the Brain Gym In-Depth One course twice and
I was interested in continuing my education,

so I took Brain Gym Masters In- Depth. From there, I really was fascinated with the In-Depth work that I was doing.

We had begun muscle testing (which will be described later in detail) during our classes and it was through this process that I found out that I needed to deal with some emotional connections in order to straighten one of my eyes out. One of the problems, caused by the paralysis, was my left eye was stuck in one position. It had always been wobbling in and out after a strabismus surgery that I had in 1966. My eye was greatly hampering my field of vision. My left eye always rolled out and had never really returned to normal. To correct this I needed to perform an Integration Metaphor (which will be described later in detail as well). During the process we spread our arms out to our sides. It took an incredible amount of strength to bring both of my hands back together to do the Integration Metaphor. You are then supposed to pull your hands apart. And an amazing thing happened. I pulled so hard and held so tight that my eye straightened out right away. This technique straightened it out immediately and I was extremely impressed with the result.

By the end of December 1994, I had completed quite a few of the Brain Gym classes. But I was still looking for other treatments and techniques that could help myself and my son. My housekeeper at the time told me that she knew someone who practiced a technique called colonics, and she asked if I would be interested in getting a treatment done. I wasn't sure what it was, but I said that I might be interested. She went on to tell me about someone who had done allergy elimination with Nambudripad Allergy Elimination technique (NAET) and it instantly piqued my interest.

She gave me the practitioner's number, and I gave the person a call. I told them that I had a son who I suspected was dealing with severe allergies and that I also had a lot of allergies myself. The woman on the phone told me that her and her husband worked together and she scheduled me an appointment with him right away. Shortly after, I went in for my first session, but I wasn't really impressed by the man that I saw. He didn't have the best bed-side manner so he came across pretty rude. He was very quick, and seemed like he wanted to get everybody out the door. His practice was like a big assembly line, and it all made me a little uncomfortable. I decided that I would tough it out and give it a try until Christmas break because my son's allergies were a big probem and I wanted to find a solution for him. I thought that if it helped him, it would be worth pushing through and really giving the technique a try. I ended up taking all four of my kids, and it started helping Nathaniel in particular.

One day, we all went in for a session, and as I was finishing, I noticed that Nathaniel was out in the waiting room running around and being crazy. That day, the practitioner was supposed to start his allergy testing, specifically with eggs. Nathaniel was very allergic to eggs, and I knew that it would be a difficult thing to test without him being able to eat them. The practitioner never did get to that test. I knew that Nathaniel required a detoxification and from there I decided to take on more of his treatment myself putting together their technique and the Brain Gym technique. I went back and talked to the people that I had been working with on the Brain Gym classes for advice and they told me about their In-depth Brain Gym class. At that time, there were about 10 people in the class, and it was a very small group from Southern California. I figured out how to get the money together and I took the class on the weekends.

I went to a few more of these sessions with the practitioners that I had been seeing. But in the end I decided that I was going to start adding my Brain Gym integration from all my Brain Gym classes that I had taken. I decided that I would just try to experiment with all of the knowledge that I had gathered to see if I could find a better solution for our health problems. I started writing down a few little things as I went. Each Brain Gym session cost quite a bit, so I figured that maybe by putting some of this together and doing it myself, I could save myself some money. I did a few more sessions and by March, I had come around. During the time that I was there, I had become friendly with a person in the office. She and I started getting together, and we started experimenting. She had been going to the NAET classes for treatment as well and she was not really comfortable with the way that they were treating patients in a sort of assembly line. So right then and there we decided we would start trying to do it ourselves. We would go to each other's houses and swap treatment back and forth, working on different areas, going through the book, and

even working on her grand children who had a
lot of allergies. We got a couple of different
books and we started experimenting with
different things, putting different
combinations together. We started working on
it, and the more we did, it sort of blossomed
and kept growing.

Meanwhile, I was still doing my Brain
Gym classes and experimenting a little bit
more on my own. I learned a lot about how
the different systems work in the body because
I had taken so many different classes. So
when we got together and we started taking
notes it just added to my knowledge . We
started going back and forth and seeing
different reactions happen with different
treatments. By that time we had both gone to
the our NAET workers a couple more times,
and we had finally gotten tired of going to the
them because of the frequency that they were
making us go. It seemed like it was every
single day we had another session. She would
have her six kids and my four, and it seemed
like we were spending most of our time in
there. We decided that wasn't very productive,
especially since it was turning into a
horrendous bill for both of us. From that
moment forward, we made a choice to do the
treatments ourselves to save ourselves some
money. Shortly after, I was trying to find a
way to get the bill down because it was getting
to be really high, so I started to work off some
of the sessions by doing some cleaning in their
office. One day, I was using my Rainbow floor
cleaner to clean the office, and I noticed these
little vials that were placed in alphabetical
order in a row. I was intrigued, and I saw a vial

for polio. I picked up the vial and I instantly started having major reactions to it. My body heat went through these seizures and I started twitching all over. I went home and I called my friend from the office. I told her what happened. While I was talking to her, I looked at myself, and my entire body started twisting and going into this seizure. I told her that she needed to come over quick to work on me. By the time she had gotten to me, which was probably five minutes or so by car, I was totally in a twisted pretzel. She was confused about what to do, so she asked me and I told her to go down my spine and check the levels (this is the Nambudripad Allergy Elimination technique) She said, "what am I supposed to do," and I said, "just keep going down my back" (this is a release technique from Nambudripad Allergy Elimination). She said, that she had never seen anybody twisted like that and started to panic a little. I said, "this is all from the polio and you have to keep going down my back, just relax and don't freak out. Don't call the paramedics because all they will do is want to give me drugs. I don't want any drugs. I just want you to keep going down my back, keep going down my back and I'll release and it will be all right." The levels unfolded as time went by and the process for healing took on a new meaning. It felt so good to be healed and feeling well again after she was done. I talked to her the next day and she said again that she had never seen anything like that. I told her that as I fought polio that most of my life had been that way. But one of the biggest takeaways from that experience was that I was extremely excited about the processes and the ability to heal it.

By word of mouth from people who saw my recovery, my business began to grow. People were beginning to use the technique that I had created and letting me work on them, and it was healing them too. I started learning about the effects that certain foods had on me, and how important clearing the allergies were. I had not been completely cleared from all of the different things from my treatments because there were so many different combinations that I had. My friend and I started at the beginning of a list of different foods, and I realized that I was very allergic to eggs. That was a very big piece for me. I started writing each allergen on little slips of paper. The one thing that I was missing was the vials with the different allergens. So I decided that I was just going to write them on a piece of paper and go down the back and do the technique just as if they were doing the procedure with the vials. One big difference between my technique and theirs is that they didn't use the different fingers to do muscle testing. But I had noticed in all of my experimenting, that when I used the different fingers, there was a big shift in the results of my testing. Each finger represented a different level or realm that the allergen needed to be processed through, and this made my technique more thorough.

My friends and I started talking and unraveling this little onion of knowledge as levels unfolded and I continued keeping notes on everything that we discovered. We started getting more and more people to work on and word of mouth started to grow. People would come, and we would work on them and very quickly I was doing this as a business. It was around this time that a couple more friends joined us in treatment. Giselle, who was a friend of mine from another Brain Gym class I had taken, and Sydney, a friend of mine who had four children. We were all very happy about getting things worked on.

My friend Giselle was very much into the different spiritual realms and universal healing. She taught me about these different realms. (Realms are specific fields of inquiry through which learning may be acquired). I started muscle checking and found out which realms we needed to work with. There were up to 48 different levels. We added metabolic, synthesis, causal, physical, spiritual, and emotional to this list. We would continue to work on these different levels, and each week we started talking about different things that we were seeing. Each level became higher and I started including quite a bit of the things that I had learned about Chinese acupressure. These were things of the five elements. Then I learned about all the different sounds and we included those. The lists that I had were very small at the beginning, and I got to muscle check in full. I would muscle check everything and kept muscle checking and muscle checking some more and I muscle checked and muscle checked and muscle checked. The greater my experience and my knowledge grew, the longer my lists would get and I would have to be more strategic about how I treated a patient because I couldn't check everything.

Everybody would call me up and ask if I could muscle check them. I would be muscle checking all the time, treating people and clearing people's blockages. By that time it was 1998 and I had gone through the beginning parts of my divorce. My life was still pretty chaotic, so we used that time to learn more about how life experiences could effect different levels and we started to discover ways to clear up different things.

In 1999, we were still very active in my Brain Gym classes and still doing all of the allergy work. As I was going through all of it and creating my technique, I didn't have a name for it quite yet. I kept calling it Brain Gym and NAET, and I didn't even know what I should call it. But very quickly I came up with the name Muscular Integrated In-Depth Therapy (MIIT).

In the year 2000 Giselle and I started to work with color and the different levels, like working on metabolic, absorption, assimilation, how the body works, and we added some color therapy. We did acupuncture and acupressure and rituals as well in combination with my own techniques. My technique evolved from just the Brain Gym and the Nambudripad Allergy Elimination techniques and became its own technique altogether. With each thing that I added, each consecutive level created even more intense shifting in patients.

It definitely has been a growing experience. Each class that I took and each person I worked on really noticed healing shifts. My name really got out there and I was really enjoying the work I was doing. But by the end of 2001, Giselle started getting ill. By April, she was diagnosed with cancer.   Her weight had been deteriorating and she had lost interest in food. We didn't know at the time that she had cancer, but we had a feeling that something wasn't quite right. By July of that same year, she had passed away. It was very sad, but we worked almost right up until she died, and we were busy. She chanted, and we did many different healing things up until the day that she died. We tried to do as much as we could while she was getting prepared. That was a wonderful transition, and it was an honor to be able to help her with that. My friend Georgia's husband also passed away from cancer that year. He wanted me to go over and help, so I worked with them – with Georgia and her family – and he passed away in April. Both Giselle and Gerry had passed away in the same year. It was a very traumatic year for us.

Work on my business continued. I spent an enormous amount of time and money learning as much as I could about the human body, allergies, phobias, emotions and feelings, etc. I did a lot of research developing this technique and as I did, I started making lists with all of the different levels on top. With the help of my nephew, I started adding more levels and the different topics so it was more organized. I got busy using the charts and that made it much easier. I must say, it has been difficult trying to get this all together, but now I'm putting it all to paper so I can share it with all of you. I have done a lot of work on this book, and as I was going through each of the different topics, I'm hopeful that it will be understandable and that everyone will be able to see how this has been a growing experience.

Now with the numbers, I have really gotten it much more fine tuned. I know exactly what each of the numbers mean so I can now be much more direct in putting my energies into the proper place where they need to go and shift things much quicker. As I did that, my treatments went from being 4 to 5 hours of work to maybe an hour, and much more intense. I did my best to be more efficient in clearing blockages without as much strain on my own body. That made it better as well. My thinking is clearer now and I am hoping that this will be able to help many people. I have created the number list and the other lists in this book to help you.

When you are working with symptoms using the MIIT system you will experience an immediate shift and notice changes as the persons body begins to integrate and their symptoms begin to decrease. Please remember to check dates and timelines of the patients experiences for accuracy (see Chapter 3 to know how to do this).

This work can be done in person [one on one] or from a distance. I myself, work with patients on the phone or via video conferencing for additional support during this integration.

I hope that through learning this technique, you will be able to not only help yourself improve your health, but that you will also be able to help countless people. Thank you for taking this journey with me.

CHAPTER 2

Introduction to Applied Kinesiology

What is Applied Kinesiology?

Applied Kinesiology (AK) is the practice of using manual muscle-strength testing for diagnosis and it can act as a tool to determine the need for subsequent treaments and what those treatments may be. According to followers of Applied Kinesiology, it works by giving feedback on the functional status of the body. AK is a practice within alternative medicine and is therefore different from "kinesiology," or the scientific study of human movement. AK draws together many similar therapies. It serves as an integrated, interdisciplinary approach to health care.

George J. Goodheart, a chiropractor, was the originator of AK in the year 1964. He developed the technique through his unique interpretation and application of Muscles: Testing and Function, which was written by two physical therapists Kendall and Kendall. Applied Kinesiology quickly spread to other chiropractors, and a few physical therapists, dentists, and medical doctors. In the year 1976, the International College of Applied Kinesiology was founded. Applied kinesiology has been used by chiropractors, naturopaths, physicians, dentists, nutritionists, physical therapists, massage therapists, nurses and more health practitioners. It is a system that evaluates structural, chemical, and mental aspects of health using a form of manual muscle testing alongside conventional diagnostic methods. The essential idea of applied kinesiology that is not shared by mainstream medical theory is that every organ dysfunction is accompanied by a weakness in a specific corresponding muscle. This is called the viscerosomatic relationship. Practitioners will then use techniques such as joint manipulation and mobilization, myofascial, cranial and meridian therapies, clinical nutrition, and dietary counseling to treat what is found in the patient through muscle testing.

A manual muscle test in AK is conducted by having the patient resist using the muscle or muscle group that is being tested while the practitioner applies a force. A smooth and locking response is sometimes called 'a strong muscle' while a response is not appropriate to proper muscle function is called 'a weak response'. This is not necessarily a test of actual muscle strength, but more of an evaluation of tension in the muscle and smoothness of the muscular response. This response of a weak muscle is considered to be an indication of stresses and imbalances within the body. A weak muscle test is related to dysfunction as well as chemical, structural imbalance, or mental stress.

The most common muscle test conducted in AK is the arm–pull–down test, or the 'Delta test'. In this test, the patient resists as the practitioner applies a downward force on an extended arm. Proper positioning of the muscle is absolutely vital in order to ensure that the muscle is isolated. Another feature of Applied Kinesiology is 'Nutrient testing'. It is used to examine the body's response to various chemicals or nutritional supplements. Taste and and smell stimulation are said to alter the outcome of a manual muscle testing. And in fact the application of the proper nutritional supplement can strengthen a weakened muscle when applied, indicating that the patient has a need for that particular nutritional supplement. Though its use frowned upon by the ICAK, testing of certain chemical/ nutritional supplements can also be done by contact with the patient (testing with the bottle of pills in the patient's hand).

Another technique used in AK is called 'Therapy localization'. It is another diagnostic technique using manual muscle testing and it is unique to applied kinesiology. In Therapy Localization, the patient places the hand of the arm which is not being tested on the skin over an area that is suspected to be in need of attention. This contact is thought to focus the mind and nervous system on the area. This leads to a change in muscle response from strong to weak or vice versa when therapeutic intervention is indicated. If the area contacted is not associated with a need for treatment, the muscle response will be unaffected.

Another use of AK is to have the subject wear colored glasses (blue, green, red, etc.) and perform the muscle testing technique while wearing each color of glasses. The color that creates the greatest smoothness of muscle response could be a color that is in some way beneficial to the client and has a positive result on their nervous system.

Supporters of the technique claim a great level of clinical efficacy. A review of the literature revealed methodological problems with previous AK studies that claimed the technique was falliable, and some studies actually do show clinical efficacy. One study showed a high degree of correlation between AK muscle testing for food allergies and antibodies for those foods. The AK procedure in this study involved stimulation of taste receptors followed by muscle testing for change in strength. The patient was suspected of being allergic to foods that disrupted muscle function. Blood drawn subsequently showed the presence of antibodies to the foods which were found to be allergenic through AK assessment. In another blinded study, the response of a calf muscle, to an inhibitory reflex technique used in AK was studied using graphical recordings of electromyography and mechanical parameters. The study found that with good coordination between the examiner and subject, muscle inhibition was easily recorded.

Some of the studies, research and reviews of applied kinesiology mentioned above are listed at the National Library of Medicine and National Institutes of Health.

American Chiropractic Association and AK

According to the American Chiropractic Association, Applied Kinesiology is the 10th most frequently used chiropractic technique in the United States. It shows that approximately 37.6% of chiropractors are employing this method and 12.9% of patients are being treated with it. The American Chiropractic Association states, 'This is an approach to chiropractic treatment in which several specific procedures may be combined. Diversified/manipulative adjusting techniques may be used with nutritional interventions, together with light massage of various points referred to as neurolymphatic and neurovascular points. Clinical decision-making is often based on testing and evaluating muscle strength.'

How Muscular Integrated In-Depth Therapy uses muscle testing and AK

Our bodies are built to endure many small traumas, and we deal with extreme compression in our daily lives, but our physical, and emotional still break down with thoughts that develop through personal experiences. And this can effect our meridian systems. As we go through some of these traumas, we experience what I call blockages in these meridians, and sometimes these blockages are connected to emotional or subconscious memories. This means that by not letting go of these past experiences, we are hurting ourselves by not letting go of the past. Even if we know of this consciously, without help, it is difficult to clear these blockages. Through muscle testing and directing the energies of the meridians learned in AK, I help clear the patient's blockages, allowing the body to become balanced in a peaceful harmony to the system. This helps individuals to achieve their highest integrated state, which allows the patient to have peace and pass through into better health in the future.

All we are is energy. Energy is created through experiences. All the generations before us are energy. Our DNA is energy. All of our thoughts and all of our memories are energy. Positive forces will make us feel good -- which in turn makes things easier to think, and easier to do. All we need to do is think positive and continue to think that way. Positive thinking is extremely important. By directing the energies in our bodies, the elements and blockages from the past can be more easily integrated.

Everything has a frequency, and all we have to do is our best to achieve peace and love through gratitude, as well as giving our bodies what they need through water and nutrients. Nutrients are essential for the body. Minerals are essential for the body. All memories, all emotions, all organs, all hormones, all systems, all neurotransmitters, time issues, different environments, and colors all affect our reality. Our reality is always changing. As we experience different events in our lives,

28

blockages can create various health problems, but through Muscular Integrated In-Depth Threrapy, blockages can be cleared and patients can feel better. That is my intention through this technique--to get people to feel better -- and I keep working to achieve this goal every day.

All of our experiences affect how we react and inter-react with other people. As we go through life, we have many things that happen and words are essential for the healing, both in how we say them and how we experience them. How people are affected by their experiences is different for everyone, but what I've experienced is that sometimes we hold these details and sometimes they interlock into our organs and make us ill. The way that I use MIIT to help this is that I take the different elements and I go through many different areas. I start on different levels. I use different meridians to check the patient's system. The meridians include but are not limited to, the essential central meridian, the vital meridian, the belt meridian, the bladder meridian, the spleen meridian, stomach meridian, and the triple warmer meridian.

Meridians: Spleen meridian, stomach large intestines, lungs, liver, regulating yen, gall bladder, vital, belt, triple warmer, circulation, sex, kidney, bladder, plexus, mobility yen, governing, central.

These meridians run through the body. They all work together as a combined unit. Each blockage released allows the indivisible stresses of the systems to be released so that new energies can flow.

All of these meridians run through our system and I redirect the meridians to let the energies leave and strengthen the system by bringing the energies higher. This allows the negative blockage energies to leave, and it strengthens the body as a result. The different levels we have are spiritual, metabolic toxins, intake, absorption, emotional, synthesis, mental, physical, integration, active, metabolism, metabolic, subconscious, conscious, cellular, ethereal, molecular, acute, actualization, time release, reality and causal. I work to remove the negative energies so the body can be strengthened and healed. In each level I check where each one is at, going through the numbers as I move along the body and muscle check different areas. As I start with my process, the numbers are usually low, which means that I haven't worked on them for whatever reason, and then we find out what each are using the Numbers list in the back (See Appendix A). The meridians being cleared brings the energies up to a thousand.

I provide this technique to serve people that want an alternative from doctors, drugs and psychologists. MIIT is a mixture of kinesiology, acupressure, massage, reflexology, and holistic care. I can, and have, helped many people to become allergy free, treat trauma, depression, post trauma stress, pain relief and vision issues.

In the next part of the book I will tell you more about how to make sure the numbers flow easily

CHAPTER 3

Explanation of Levels and how they work

Introduction to MIIT

In order to teach you this technique, I need to first explain to you how I arrive at the levels and how to properly conclude what is going on with the patient. The levels are the numbers that represent the causes (in a metaphorical sense) of the main problem that a client presents to me. So as carefully explained as possible, here is my process for finding the levels.

When I meet a client, I first sit for a few minutes to clear myself. I do not want to make eye contact with the client, because I want to focus on their problem and not on their person. I don't want any distractions. I then ask them what issue they want to focus on. The issue or the concern of the person is called the TOPIC (ie, diabetes, insomnia, addictions, allergies, and emotional issues such as depression, grief, and lack of joy.) They may only have symptoms and aren't sure yet what the topic is. In which case, I may need to ask questions and get a history to figure out what they are asking for specifically. After I find the topic, I need to find the underlying cause of the topic. The cause is the level. The cause (hereafter called the level) has a number that I find using applied kinesiology (also known as muscle testing). This system of levels is what I call the MIIT Muscle Checking Number System (MCNS).

I should explain how I arrive at the number that represents the level. The way I count is by putting a finger on my left hand together with the tip of my thumb (like I was making a circle with my fingers) and then using my right index finger, I lightly grab my left thumb and tug. I am looking for a "lock". This is when my right index "grabs' the circle on the left hand and doesn't break the circle (watch the video on my website – MarijaneLeacroartIIT.org to see exactly how I do it). This 'lock' would be answering a question in the affirmative. If your index finger breaks the circle, the question is answered in the negative. When the question is answered in the negative, that is the determinant of where the issue is. Which finger I use will depend on the realm (to use Paul Dennison's term) that the level is in. The explanation for each fingers representation can be found in the next section.

I start by using the above referenced technique on my index finger, which represents the physical realm. If the circle breaks, I use the technique with the next finger. This will indicate if the level is in the emotional realm. If the circle breaks, I go to the third finger, which will show me if it is in the spiritual realm. If that finger doesn't lock, I use the technique with the pinkie finger. If the circle holds, then the level is in the acu realm, which is a term from Paul Dennison. Essentially, whichever finger I find a lock in will be the realm that the problem is in. Once I find the realm, I can find the level.

Finding the Level (Number):

To find the level, I use the same finger technique using the finger representing the realm, but I start counting. I start counting at 1 and count all the way up until I feel a lock. The cause (or level) is found when I reach the number that represents the level and the circle made by the fingers hold, or 'lock.' Once I have the number of the cause, I then use the same applied kinesiology technique I explained above to find how many blockages there are. If I get a lock (ie the circle holds) on 0, the blockage is going to be represented by a negative number. That means that the block is big. The goal is to move the blockages until I get 1000. If I get 0, I count backwards. Most of the time, the 'lock' doesn't happen on 0 and the numbers are positive. In that more common situation, I count from 1 to 10, then count 20, 30, 40, up to 100, all the while looking for a 'lock' using the applied kinesiology muscle testing technique. Let's say I get a lock on 40. I will then know my number is between 40 and 50, so I will count 41, 42, 43 etc. If I don't get a 'lock' by 100, I continue counting 100, 200, 300 etc. I, for example, might get a lock on 600, and then I start counting 610, 620 etc. And the previous method of counting by 10's applies.

In this process, I will get a series of numbers that represent blockages or contributing factors to the level of the topic. If there are many factors, there will be many numbers.

Finding the Associated Letter:

Once I have the series of numbers, I find the contributing factors, which I call a subtitle. The subtitle can be found using the same applied kinesiology technique (using the same finger/realm throughout) by going through the alphabet starting at 'A.' When I get a 'lock' on a particular letter, I use the applied kinesiology technique to find the word that represents the subtitle. For instance, if I get a lock on 'l,' I go through words that start with 'l' in the **'Questions list'**. If I get a lock on a word in the questions list then that is an affirmative response. If I do not get a lock on a word in the **'Questions' list**, then I will start going down alphabetically through the emotions list, looking for a lock.

Finding the Associated Date:

Once I find the subtitle, I find the date associated with it. The date can be found using the same muscle checking technique and the list in the 'how time is used in integration' section of this book. Starting with the first letter of the month, moving to the day and then the year. If it is relevant, I might get a lock on a time too. I will know if it is relevant by asking 'is there a time that I should look for?' This date might refer to a trauma in this life or a past life. Occasionally, it has something to do with a future life, but that is rare. This date represents a memory that my client associates with something related their topic. I always ask at this point, "Is this all?" Or "Do I have all the information that I need to clear all the blockages?" and use the applied kinesiology technique. If the fingers lock, then I have all the information that I need. If not, I have to do more muscle checking for subtitles. When I have all the information, I use the integration metaphor, which I explain in another section of this book.

Compared to an Outline with Different Topic & Subtopic

Using the MIIT Individual worksheet,(we will call our subject "Tim"), we will attempt to explain the process of revealing the blockages and the level at which they currently are in the columns labeled Toxins, Integration and Active.

Example; His Topic is Need for more Spirituality in his life. #97 (Keytones, Sweetness of Life) from the list of 100 (List can be found in the next section) .

On the left is 9 and on the right is 7 (the number 97 is split into two separate numbers, reading left (on the left hemisphere of the brain) and right (on the right hemisphere of the brain.)

On the right- Number 9 is Copper (from the MCNS)
On the left – Number 7 is Opinion (from MCNS)

Starting on the right Copper, look for how many blockages are stopping "Tim" from achieving his highest potential by using the MCNS.

There may be 17 (17 is Crushed) of these (ie. muscle, hydration, emotions).

Starting on the Left Opinion, check for how many blockages are stopping "Tim" by using the MCNS. There may be 31 (Hopelessness)

This is 3 and 1. 3 is Worth and 1 is Corn. Check for blockages under 3 and one.

= 1=Corn/Behavior

SAMPLE TOPIC

Topic is Ear

By muscle checking #19 is found, which is
Mold 19 Mold

4 Chicken fat (hearing) Communication 6
Persistent

2 Assault

19 + 4=194 Corn, Urenic Acid (deals with
feelings–lymph) Belief Systems 4 + 6=
Analytical–thinking too much, over–focused

2 + 6= Fibular collateral ligament (stepping
forward into the future 19, 4, 6, 2, 26, 46, 194
(1, 94)

Up = positive number

Down= negative number (chronic or causal–
has been around a long time, ie. –Past Life

Personal Worksheet for Tim (Example)

Different Levels (Realms)–Networks of
information from the brain through finger/
thumb circuits. The finger modes are realm
indicators.

First Finger (Pointer) - Structure/Movement Realm

ORANGE
Toxins – A poisonous substance. It has
a protein structure secreted by certain
organisms and capable of causing toxicities
when introduced into the body tissues. It is
also capable of inducing a counteragent or an
antitoxin. 16
Integration – The act of merging or growing
into each other in a series of stages, forms or
types. 26
Active– Causing or initiating action or change.
2

YELLOW
Causal– Expressing or indicating cause. 62
Physical– having material existence;
perceptible especially through the senses and
subject to the laws of nature. 4 6 Up
Actualization– Existing in fact or reality. 6 12
Up
Molecular – Of or relating to simple or
elementary organization. 30 9 Up
Intake– That which is taken in; especially,
energy taken in. 9 7 Up
Expressive Arts – Integrated Movements and
Issues Drawing, Movement Dance, Writing,
Role play, Resonation
Resonate laugh, sing, cry, sigh, shout
Receptive Process – Anchor (RNA Point), Transforma-
tional Vehicle (Cook's Hook- Ups, Positive Pts, Light,
Neurovasculars), Issue (Affirmative statement) Age (Past
memory, Future
Construct), Support (Supportive Touch, Eye Activation,
Guilded Visualization, Integrating Music)

Astral- 100 21 Up
Structural- 4 11 Up

Second Finger (Middle) - Personal Ecology Realm
GREEN
Metabolism- the complex of physical
and chemical processes involved in the
maintenance of life. 29 9 Up Page 824
Spiritual- concerned with or affecting the soul.
45 3 Up
but exists necessarily. 72 12 Up
Spiritual Memory 410
Atomic- existing in the state of separate
atoms. 43 2 Up
Reality - something that is neither derivative
nor dependent

Third Finger (Ring) - Emotional Realm

BLUE
Emotional - Agitation of the passions or
sensibilities often involving physiological
changes. Any strong feeling such as joy,
sorrow, reverence, hate, or love. These arise
subjectively rather than through conscious
mental effort. 38
Ethereal - Of or relating to the regions beyond
the world. 57
Mental - Of or relating to the mind; response
of or relating to the total emotional and
intellectual response of an individual to his
environment. 8 8 Up
Absorption- To take in through or as through
pores or interstices; soak in or up 49
Penia (Chi)- Life force energy 904 Body, brain
+ action- 908 Thought process: Body/Brain

Check all angles
Point of impact
Evidence – In its broadest sense includes everything that is used to determine or demonstrate the truth of an assertion.
Summary – The summary has 6 blocks of 2 distinct numbers. For example: (12,13) (14,15) (6,17) (118,19) (20,21) (22,23) This summarizes the issue. Each digit corresponds to an Integrate In-Depth Therapy value. See the word and number lists. Neurolymphatic points
Neurovascular points
Host Patterns
Details
Issues
Experience
Auditory processing
Frequency

Fourth Finger (pinky) - Acu-Realm

PURPLE
Subatomic– Of, or relating to the inside of the atom or to particles smaller than atoms. 28
Time release– Time– A continuum which lacks spatial dimensions and in which event succeed one another from past through present to future. 12
Release – To relieve from something that confines, burdens or oppresses. Synthesis – The production of a substance by the union of chemical elements, groups or simpler compounds by the degradation of a complex compound. 32
Metabolic (METAMORPHOSIS)– Pertaining to or undergoing metamorphosis. 84 Up Page

824
Spiritual Memory 410 (13 metabolic) 9 Up 32 level
Extreme core 59
Assimilation– Absorb as nourishment/ understand 83
Chronic– Always present or encountered 11
Acute – Responsive to slight impressions or stimuli. 903
Reonia – Chemical reaction that deals within the brain 908
Cellular– Of, relating to, or consisting of cells 33
Conscious – Perceiving, apprehending, or noticing with a degree of controlled thought or observation, social – ie: **Group consciousness** (church, support group, people of same belief)– 12
Subconscious 5
Social (Weather) (Rain) – 81,
Intention 1000
Core of body Shoulder of shoulder Hip to hip

Base
Inside (healing circle)
Outside (healing circle)
Together
Split
Recheck
Core / output
Reflexes
Focus
Visualization
Universe pose– Fingers of each hand touching tips of corresponding fingers of the other hand. Dealing with the higher level of consciousness

(astral) and earthly experience (space, planets, other worlds). 79

During treatment, you will be referring to a number of lists that can be found in Appendix A in the back of this book. Every patient and every treatment will be different, but it is very important that you take your time, be patient, and persistent to work through and clear every level of blockage.

CHAPTER 4

Integration

Integration Metaphor (IM)

The word Integration as defined by Paul Denison PhD in his Vision Circles Handbook (p. 60) is the lifelong process of realizing ones physical, mental, and spiritual potential, the first step being the simultaneous activation of both cerebral hemispheres for specific learning; the act or process of making whole; or complete.

The word metaphor comes from the Greek word metapherien, meaning to transfer. Meta involving change and pherein meaning to bear. Denison also describes the following: "Denison Laterality Re-patterning* The Brain Gym

Handbook (p. 20) is not suggested as a panacea for all our ills. One of the first steps of any sound educational or health maintenance program. It is providing results for people who have failed to find help elsewhere. It is literally true, as many are learning that we must crawl before we walk". The integration metaphor that is used is comparing the 54 Levels or layers of energy to an onion or an artichoke. This is used to describe how a person begins to heal in layers. As he/she heals he literally peels through the different blockages to the sweeter "heart" of life. this brings him/her to Sweetness of Life which is Ketones (# 97 of the MIIT Muscle Checking Number System (MCNS).

The corpus callosum is the structure connecting the two sides of the brain. It contains the neurotransmitters which communicate between the right and left sides of the brain. The Integration Metaphor, used with the MIIT In-Depth Levels and Muscle Checking can strengthen the corpus callosum and assists in integrating by pulling the intention (energy) directing each level and bringing both the right and left hemispheres of the brain to full fruition. This is an excellent tool for intention. Used with the In-Depth Levels and Finger Muscle Checking, it assists integration by pulling the intention (energy) directing each level. IM can also be used with phone work from a distance, this is an excellent tool for intention.. Used in combination with MIIT it can speed up the integration of the healing process.

How the IM is done is as follows:

The thumbs of each hand touch a finger of
the same hand forming a ring or circle. The
thumb represents the heart. The fingers represent. When this ring is formed the arms are
extended and then brought together to cross
each other. These are then brought towards the
heart with deep intention.

A 5 Step process –

1. Cross crawl
2. Lateral Crawl
3. The Integration Metaphor
4. Cross crawl
5. Homolateral crawl while thinking of an x.

How an Energy Blockage Effects the Body:

An energy that is not allowing the body to
achieve its highest potential. It can affect the
body by having pain, raise blood pressure or
blood sugar level. Each and every blockage
must be cleared with each topic or (goal) to see
the complete and full evidence. The topic
has to be specific and detailed. Some change
may be evident as blockage energies are lifted
along the way by a behavior change. Total
integration may take full level and Meridian clearing. A blockage can be minor or major with many issues, areas, angles, options,
dates and events. Address all combinations.
Opportunities, experiences, traumas and dra-
mas can compound and appear make a new

Proper placement:

The order of importance
Tracing treatment
Smell / olfactory
Touch/proprioceptor
Important for body order communication graphs vision
Record keeping
Hearing: color/tunes/music

To Clear Meridians:

It is important in choosing a topic or goal to ask questions that all add up to 100%. When you have the details, you are able to assist the Blockage to be free to leave with few or no reactions. The reaction does not need to be dramatic to be positive. Positive changes are better and easy to understand. Each system can be simple.

From a minute to up to a month or year you will begin to see evidence that can be subtle or remarkable.

What is an Allergy?

An abnormal reaction of the body to a previously encountered allergen introduced by inhalation, ingestion, injection, drugs, skin contact, often manifested by itchy eyes, runny nose, wheezing, skin rash, or diarrhea.

What is an Allergen?

An allergen is a substance that in some persons induces the hypersensitive state of allergy and stimulates the formation of reaginic antibodies. Allergens may be naturally occurring or of synthetic origin and include pollen, mold spores, dust, animal dander, insect debris, foods, blood serum, and drugs. Identification of allergens is made by studying both the site of symptoms (ie. inhalants such as molds, pollens, and dander usually effect the eyes, nose and bronchi...cosmetics often effect the skin of the face and hands) and the time that symptoms appear (ie., seasonal allergy to pollen). Allergens caused by foods like corn and grasses can cause skin reddening. If they are not cleared these can go deeper into our system and affect bones, nerves, muscles, organs, etc.

Allergens come in 7 Categories:

1. Inhalents
2. Ingestants
3. Contactants
4. Injectants
5. Molds
6. Fungi
7. Physical Agents

The level on the physical is what we see but all the levels are affected by the allergens. I use the numbers to track your progress since it isn't always obvious that something has changed after the allergy has been dealt with.

Questions to ask when you or another person is reacting

Muscle check the following items by asking "where each is at"(where it is at on toxins, integration or active). Keep in mind that the reaction may be a delayed reaction. These may have happened on the day of the visit, or recently.

This is your personal choice. This is not meant to replace them but it is your body – your life.

The following are things to check:

· What was eaten.

· Inhaled.

· Touched

· What was heard.

· Seen or witnessed.

· People they came in contact with.

· Things they read.

· Things felt today.

· Any and all conversations had (ask whether in person or by telephone, internet, video con-ferencing etc.) that may have a had a negative effect on them.

· Any assaults by persons today (this would actually fall under the category of persons to whom you or your client has had contact with).

· Any dreams had last night or recently that you believe may have a barring on what is happening now.

· All biological agents they have been exposed to.

· All chemicals they may have been exposed to.

· All bodily functions and processes.

· All bodily produced toxins (i.e. skatol, indole, etc)

· All bodily other substances (such as hormones, neurotransmitters, enzymes, etc.). Doctor provided or otherwise.

· All devices this person have come in contact with (electronic or mechanical that are new or different).

· All substances they think my have been inhaled (such as mold spores – in a lot of dwellings and you may not know are there). Everything ingested recently (different than ate --- as in conscious vs. unconscious of substance).

As I have worked on my technique, I have found that all things are connected. I learned that 20 different genes are involved in determining immune system function. T-helper 1- cell, T-helper-2-cells become more active with allergenic foods such as eggs, corn, etc, long after sensitization, thus releasing IGE to the specific allergen. It is essential to clear IGE levels. These are listed to clear in order of importance:

*Proper Placement

*Smell/Olfactory

*Tastants
       -Taste receptors send messages to the hypo thalamus region of the brain.

*Hormones

How History & Time is Part of Integration

Time cells: (Past,Past) – (Past, Present) – (Past, Future) – (Present,Past) – (Present, present) –

(Present, Future) – (Future, Past) – (Future,Future) Dates: Month – Day-Year | Time: a.m. – p.m.

January–,Febuary–,March–,April,–May,–June–July,August,September,October,November,December,– 1,2,3,4,5,6,7,8,9,10,11,12,13,14,15,16,17,18,19,20,21,22,2324,25,26,27,28,29,30,31

Past,,,Present Beliefs,,,Life Beliefs,,,Future Goals Past Lives:

Age regeneration, present back with past year example 1800–1700 or 1700–1600, etc.1800's ask for specific date.

Present perception of beliefs: How would you see yourself without this block? Future Goals: What is integration? Webster says:

'Coordination of mental processes into a normal effective personality or with an individual's environment.'

How the body receives and acknowledges the information. How long will it take to integrate into my body? It depends on the individual and how severe the condition is.

The following are questions to ask and things to check for when muscle-checking (testing) for various factors affecting a topic

Ask how many of these things and in some cases, the What and the Who. These are meant to help "shift" the energy when raising the frequency level of a topic.

Of course, many below can become topics --- when discovered in an of themselves.

A

ABBERATIONS

ABUSES
- Emotional
- Physical
- Mental
- From Parents
- From Siblings
- Relatives
- Sexual Abuses

ACIDS
- phytic acid
- anthocyanins
- citric acid
- ascorbic acid
- lipoic acid
- lactic acid
- fatty acids
- uric acid
- formic acid
- carbonic acid
- carbolic acid
- phosphoric acid
- pyruvic acid
- propanoic acid
- malic acid
- tartaric acid
- oxalic acid
- salicyclic acid
- acetic acid
- butyric acid
- panthothenic acid
- ethanoic acid

- boric acid
- hydrochloric acid
- nitric acid
- hydroflouric acid
- sulfuric acid
- carboxylic acid
- ethanoic acid
- trichloroethanoic acid
- amino acids
- sulfonic acid
- D–glucuronic acid
- neo acids

ANIMALS

ATTITUDES

ALLERGIES

ASSAULTS

ASTRAL INFLUENCES

AMINO ACID

These are the chemicals that combine in a variety of ways in order to make proteins. Some of them you already make, and some you have to eat in order to stay healthy. The last are called essential amino acids. For some reason, I often find that I have to remove people's sensitivity issues to amino acids, so here is a list that you might need clearing.

- Cysteine
- Taurine
- Tyrosine

- Histidine
- Leucine
- Lysine
- Isoleucine
- Arginine
- Tryptophan
- Phenylalanine
- Glycine
- Threonine
- Alanine
- Valine
- Glutamic acid
- Proline
- Asparagine
- Serine

AUTHORITATIVE FIGURES

ARCHETYPES
- Martyr

ADDICTION
- Sexual
- Drug
- Gambling
- Emotional
- Physical (OCD's)
- Food

B

BEATS
- Rhythms
- Patterns

- Stripes
- Polka Dots
- Mosaics
- Repeat units of patterns

BELIEFS
- Subconscious
- Conscious

BETRAYALS

BLOCKS
- Emotional
- Mental
- Casual
- Etheric
- Spiritual

BLOOD TOXINS

BLOWN OPPORTUNITY

BODILY SYSTEMS
- Skeletal
- Muscular
- Circulatory
- Autonomic Nervous System
- Central Nervous System
- Sympathetic Nervous System

BOTCHED DEALS

BRAIN PARTS
- See Chapter 6

BREAKDOWN OF SUPPORTS

C

CARES

CHALLENGES

CHEMICALS

COGNITIVE DISSONANCE

COLORS
- Hues
- Values
- Contrast

CONCERNS
- Personal
- Family
- Political
- Environmental
- Economic
- Spiritual

CONCUSSIONS

CONFUSED ENERGIES

CONFUSIONS

CONVERSATIONS

CORDS
- Attachments to others
- Others attachments to us
- Check friends, others

CREDITS

CRISIS

D

DATES
- Future dates
- Day/month/year/time/am/pm

DEBTS
- Personal
- Financial
- Business
- Family

DEBITS
- From 'cell bank account (greater the debit, the weaker the cell becomes—see pg. 17 of 'Why people don't heal and how they can by Caroline Myss—example—holding onto negative events from the past depletes our cellular bank accounts

DECISIONS
- Good or bad (relative to individual)

DEGREE IN WHICH NOT LIVING IN THE PRESENT MOMENT

DENSITIES OF MATTER

DEPRESSIONS OR DEPRESSIVE EPI-SODES

DEVASTATIONS

DEVIATIONS

DIALOG

DIMENSIONS

DISCLOSURES

DISCONTENTMENTS

DISEASES
- Acute conditions
- Chronic
- Iatrogenic
- Inherited disorders

DYSFUNCTIONS
- Physical
- Mental
- Emotional

E

ELEMENTALS
- Wind
- Earth
- Fire
- Water

ELEMENTS
- Carbon
- Sulfur
- Hydrogen
- Oxygen
- Hydrogen Peroxide

EMOTIONS

EMPATHIES

ENCROACHMENTS

ENERGIES

ENSLAVEMENTS
- Psychic enslavements
- Enteric
- By devices
- By mind control

ENVIRONMENT
- Home
- Physical
- Social
- Thoughts

ENZYMES

EVENTS
- Personal
- Town
- City
- State
- National
- World
- Province

EXPERIENCES
- Physical
- Psychic
- Spiritual
- Universal
- Personal
- Worldly
- Otherworldly

F

FABRICS

FAILED RELATIONSHIPS

FAILURES

FEARS
- Of Success
- Of Failure

FEELINGS OF OBLIGATION

FIRST IMPRESSIONS

FOODS

FREQUENCIES
- Hz (Hertz)
- kHz (kilohertz)
- MHz (megahertz)
- GHz (gigahertz)
- THz (terahertz)
- One hertz simply means 'one cycle per second' (typically that which is being counted is a complete cycle). 100 Hz means 'one hundred cycles per second' and so on.

FRUSTRATIONS

G

GALAXIES

GLANDS

'GONE SOUR DEALS'
- Failed agreements

GRUDGES

GUILTS

H

HABITS
HAUNTED

HARASSMENTS

HEALINGS

HEAVY METALS

HURTS

HYPNOSES
· Subliminal messages

I

INCONSISTENCIES
· Not doing and living what you believe

INFATUATIONS

INFRACTIONS

INHALANTS

INHUMANE ACTS

INJURIES

INJUSTICES

INSECURITIES

ISSUES

INVASIONS

J

JEOPARDIES

JUDGEMENTS

K

KARMIC PIECES

L

LEGENDS

LESIONS

LEVELS

LEVELS OF REALITY

LIFE LESSONS

LOSSES

LOVE

LOYALTIES

M

MATERIALS READ

MENTAL

- Emotional
- Past life
- Present life

MENTAL DISTURBANCES

MENTAL STATES

MELVIN

MEMORIES

- PRESENT LIFE
- Conscious memories
- Subconscious memories
- PAST LIFE
- Conscious life
- Subconscious life

MERIDIANS

MESSAGES

- Subliminal
- Otherwordly
- Subconscious
- From childhood
- From dreams
- From adulthood experiences
- Societal

MIND CONTROL

MINERALS

- Trace minerals

MISCONCEPTIONS

MOLDS

MOTIVATIONS

N

NEGATIVE SPIRITS
- Entities
- Dark forces

NEUROTRANSMITTERS

NOT LETTING GO OF NEGATIVE EVENTS IN THE PAST
- A refusal to move on–whether it be conscious or not

O

OBJECTS

OBSESSIONS
- With objects
- With people
- With places
- With things
- With sounds
- With acts
- With tastes
- With sights
- With thoughts

OBSTRUCTIONS

OFFENSES
- To others
- To self
- Inflicted upon self by others

OF 'LACK' OF CONSCIOUSNESS

OPPORTUNITIES

OUTBURSTS

P

PAST LIVES

PAINFUL EPISODES

PARASITES

PATHOGENS
- Viruses
- Bacteria
- Retrovirus
- Nanobacteria

PEOPLE
- Relatives
- Friends
- Enemies

PHOBIAS

- Arachnophobia
- Acrophobia
- Aerophobia
- Agoraphobia
- Brontophobia
- Carcinophobia
- Cat Phobia
- Caligynephobia
- Claustrophobia
- Clown Phobia
- Dendrophobia
- Dog Phobia
- Driving Phobia
- Enochiophobia
- Erythrophobia
- Emoetophobia
- Glossophobia
- Hydrophobia
- Necrophobia
- Needle Phobia
- Nudophobia
- Olfactophobia
- Ornithophobia
- Podophobia
- Pupaphobia
- Social Phobia
- Thanatophobia
- Trichophobia
- Zoophobia

PLACES

PLANETS

PRESSURES

R

RADIATIONS
- EMF
- Cellular phone
- HAARP–High Frequency Active Auroral Research Program
- EISCAT–European Incoherent Scatter Association Microwaves
- ELF–Extremely low frequency
- Nuclear

RADIOACTIVE HEAVY METALS

RECONCILIATIONS
- Gone sour ones

RECOURSES

REFLEXES
- Moro
- Juvenile suck
- Rooting
- Palmar
- Spinal Galant
- Gait
- Stepping and Heel
- Infant Plantar
- Hand Gait
- Babinski
- Vestibularocular Motor
- Asymmetrical Tonic Neck
- Fear Paralysis
- Tonic Labyrinthine
- Symmetrical Tonic Neck
- Suprapubic

RELATIONSHIPS

RELIGIOUS CONVICTION

RESENTMENT

RIDICULES

RITUALS

RULERS

S

SACRIFICES

SCENTS

SELF-INFLICTIONS

SELF-PITIES

SENSITIVITIES

SHACKLES AND THAT WHICH HAM-PERS US IN ANY MANNER

SHOCKS

SHORT-COMINGS

SITUATIONS

SMOTHERING
- Toward others
- Of others toward the person

T

TESTS
- Spiritual
- Mental
- Psychological
- Emotional
- Psychic
- Physical
- Academic

THOUGHTS

TIME ZONES

TONES
- Octaves
- Notes
- Discordant sounds
- Harmonic sounds
- Note combinations

TOXIC BEHAVIORS
- Example of women wearing age-inappropriate clothes or a man driving a hot red sports car into his late retirement years–it is NOT letting go of the past (Lupus is tied directly to fear of letting go).

TOXIC RELATIONSHIPS

TRAGEDIES

TRAUMAS
- In vitro
- Physical
- Psychic
- Psychological

U

UNIVERSES

V

VAGARIES

VICTORIES

VIEWPOINTS

VITAMINS

VIOLATIONS

VIOLATIONS UPON OTHERS

W

WONDER

WORRIES

WOUNDS

Y

YEASTS

CHAPTER 5

Feelings and Actions

A List of Feelings and Actions

A lot of emotions can come up when you are working on a client. It can be helpful to have a list of feelings and actions that you can run down and see if they need to be cleared. Be aware that while checking these things, the client can become emotional. Just remember to be patient and compassionate while they work through it.

I muscle check for things in this list if a client is making difficult decisions. I first ask what feeling or action will help to speed up the client's integrations with a date that I have already discovered using the muscle checking system (See page 49). I go down the list and muscle check each word using the muscle testing technique I described earlier in the book.

When the date and feeling or act are cleared together, the change should be faster and easier than if they were done on different days. Treat the fun word list the same way as the Feelings and Actions list, except that these words are not paired with dates and they are done in a separate treatment for a more upbeat response.

A LIST OF FEELINGS AND ACTIONS

A

abandoned	abused
abashed	abysmal
abducted	abyssal
aberrant	accelerated
aberration	acceptable
abhorred	accepted
abject	accepting
ablaze	accessible
able	accident prone
abnormal	acclaimed
abominable	acclimated
above average	accomodated
abrasive	accommodating
absent-minded	accomplished
absolved	accosted
absorbed	accosting
absorbent	accountable
abstemious	accredited
abstract	accurate
absurd	accused
abstracted	accusatory
abulic	accusing

acerbic
aching
acknowledged
acquiescent
acquisitive
acrimonious
activated
active
actualized
accurate
adamant
addicted
adept
adequate
admirable
admiration
admired
admiring
admonished
adorable
adored
adoring
adorned
adrift
adroit
adult
adulterated
advanced
adventurous
adverse
affable
affected
affection
affectionate
affirmed
afflicted
affluent

affray
affrayed
affronted
aflutter
afraid
against
agape
aggravated
aggressive
aggrieved
aghast
agitated
aglow
agnostic
agog
agonized
agony
agoraphobic
agreeable
ahead
ail
ailed
aimless
airy
alarmed
alcoholism
alert
alien
alienated
alive
allied
allowed
allowing
allured
alluring
alone
aloof

almighty
alright
altruistic
amateur
amazed
amazing
ambiguous
ambitious
ambivalent
ambushed
amenable
amiable
amorous
amused
amusing
analyzed
anarchistic
anchored
anemic
anesthetized
angry
angst
angsty
anguish
anguished
anhedonia
animated
animosity
annihilated
annoyed
annoying
anonymous
apathetic
apprehensive
antagonistic
antagonized
anticipation

antiquated
antisocial
antsy
anxiety
anxious
apart
apathetic
apathy
apologetic
apologized to
appalled
appealing
appeased
applauded
appraised
appreciated
appreciative
apprehension
apprehensive
approachable
appropriate
approved of
aquiver
archaic
ardent
argued with
argumentative
aristocratic
aroused
arrogant
artful
articulate
artificial
artistic
artless
ascetic
ashamed

asinine
asleep
asocial
asphyxiated
assaulted
assertive
assessed
asunder
assuaged
assured
astonished
astounded
astute
asymmetrical
at a loss
at ease
at home
at peace
at peril
at rest
at risk
at war
atrocious
atrophied
attached
attacked
attentive
attracted
attractive
atypical
audacious
austere
authentic
authoritarian
authoritative
autocratic
automated
automatic
available
avaricious
avenged
average
avid
avoided
awake
awakened
aware
awe
awed
awesome
awestruck
awful
awkward
awry

B

babied
babyish
backward
bad
bad-tempered
badgered
baffled
baited
balanced
ballistic
bamboozled
banal
banished
bankrupt
banned
bantered
bare

barracked
barraged
barred
barren
base
bashful
battered
battle-weary
battle-worn
bawled out
bearable
bearish
beastly
beat
beaten
beaten down
beatific
beautiful
beckoned
bedazzled
bedeviled
bedraggled
befriended
befuddled
beginning
beggarly
begged
beguiled
behind
beholden
beleaguered
belittled
bellicose
belligerent
belonging
below average
beloved

bemused
bemoaning
benevolent
benign
bent
berated
bereaved
bereft
beseeched
berserk
beset
besieged
besmirched
besotted
bestial
betrayed
better
bewildered
bewitched
bewitching
biased
big
bilious
binding
blinders on
bitched at
bitchy
biting
bitter
bizarre
black
black hole
being in one
blackened
blacklisted
blackmailed
blah

blame-free
blamed
blameless
blaming
bland
blank
blanketed
blasphemous
blasted
bleak
bled
bleeding
blending
blew it
blighted
blind
bliss
blissful
blithe
blocked
bloody
bloody-minded
bloomed
blooming
blossomed
blossoming
blown-apart
blown around
blown away
blown to bits
blown to pieces
blown up
bludgeoned
blue
blur
blurred
blurry

boastful
bodacious
boggled
bogus
boiling
boisterous
bold
bombarded
bombastic
bondage
bonkers
bordering
bored
boring
bossed-around
bossy
bothered
bothersome
bought
bouncy
bound
bound-up
boxed-in
bowled-over
braced
brainwashable
brainwashed
brainy
bragging
brash
bratty
brave
brazen
breathless
breathtaking
breezy
brindled

bright
bright eyed
bright eyed and bushy tailed
brilliant
brisk
bristling
broken
broken-hearted
broken down
broken-up
brooding
broody
browbeaten
bruised
brushed-off
busted
brutal
brutalized
brutalish
bubbly
bucky
bugged
buggered
building
bullied
bullish
bullshitted to
bummed
bummed out
buoyant
burdened
burdensome
buried
burned
burned-out
burned up
bursting

bushed
bushwacked
busy
buzzed
bypassed

C

caged
cajoled
calculating
callous
callow
calm
calmed down
cannibalized
canny
cantankerous
capable
capitulated
capitulating
capitulation
capricious
captious
captivated
captivating
captive
captured
cared about
cared for
carefree
careful
careless
careworn
caring
carried away

cast about
cast out
castigated
catapulted
catatonic
categorized
catty
caught
cautious
cavalier
censored
censured
centered
certain
chafed
chagrined
chained
challenged
challenging
changed
changing
chaotic
charged
charismatic
charitable
charmed
charming
charlatan
chased
chaste
chastised
chatty
cheap
cheapened
cheated
cheated on
cheeky
cheerful
cheerless
cheery
cherished
chic
chicken
chided
childish
childless
childlike
chilled
chipper
chivalrous
choked
choked-up
chosen
chucked out
chuffed
churlish
circumspect
circumvented
civil
civilized
classy
claustrophobic
clean
cleansed
clear
clear-headed
clenched
clever
clingy
cloistered
close
closed
closed in
closed-minded

clouded

compatible

cloudy

coped with

clowned (made a fool of)

compelled

clued in

competent

clueless

competitive

clumsy

copied

clung to

coping

coarse

complacent

coaxed

complaining

cocky

complete

codependent

complex

coddled

compliant

coerced

complicated

cold

complementary

cold-blooded

complimented

cold-hearted

complimentary

collapsed

composed

collapsing

compressed

collected

compromised

colonized

compromising

colorful

compulsive

comatose

compunction

combative

conceited

comfortable

concentrated

comforted

concerned

comfy

condemned

commanded

condescended-to

commanding

condescending

committed

confident

common

confined

commonplace

confirmed

communicative

confirming

companionship

conflicted

comparative

conforming

compared

confounded

copasetic

confronted

compassionate

confronting

confrontive
confused
congenial
connected
conned
conniving
conquered
conscientious
conscious
consecrated
conservative
considerate
considered
consistent
consoled
consoling
conspicuous
consulted
consumed
contagious
contained
contaminated
contemplative
contempt
contemptible
contemptuous
content
contented
contentious
contrary
contradictory
contributing
convinced
convincing
cool
cooperative
copasetic

coping
cordial
cornered
corralled
correct
corrosive
corrupt
corrupted
counterfeit
courage
cowardly
coy
cozy
crabby
crafty
cramped
cranky
crap
crappy
crass
craving
crazed
crazy
creeped out
creepy
creative
credulous
criticized
cross
crossed
cross-examined
crotchety
crowded
crucified
cruddy
crude
cruel

crummy
crumpled
crushed
crying
cultivated
cultured
cumbersome
cunning
cupidity
curious
curmudgeonly
cursed
cut
cut-down
cute
cut-off
cynical

D

dalliance
damned
dangerous
dared
daring
dark
dashed
dashing
daunted
dauntless
dazed
dazzled
dead
dear
debased
debated

debauched
debilitated
decadent
deceitful
deceptive
decided
decimated
decrepit
dedicated
defamed
deafened
defeated
defective
defenseless
defensive
deferent
defiant
deficient
defiled
definite
dehumanized
dejected
delayed
deleted
deleterious
delicate
delighted
delightful
delinquent
delirious
delivered
deluded
demanding
demeaned
denial
dependency
deprived

depressed
derided
demented
demolished
denatured
denigrated
denounced
dense
denatured
dependable
depended upon
dependent
depleted
deported
depraved
deprecated
depreciated
depressed
deprived
derailed
derided
derisive
desecrated
deserted
deserving
desiccated
desirable
desire
desired
desirous
desolate
despair
despairing
desperate
despicable
despised
despondent

destitute
destroyed
destructive
desultory
detached
detestable
detested
detoxified
devalued
devastated
deviant
devilish
devious
devoid
devoid of...
devoted
devoured
devout
diagnosed
dictated to
dictatorial
different
difficult
dim
dimensionless
diminished
diminutive
diplomatic
dire
direct
directionless
dirty
disabled
disaffected
disagreeable
disappointed
disappointing

disapproved of
disapproving
disbelieved
discomfit
discombobulated
disconcerted
disconnected
disconsolate
discontent
discontented
discounted
discouraged
discredited
discriminated
discriminating
discreet
disdain
disdained
disdainful
disembodied
dis empowered
disenchanted
disfavored
disgraced
disgruntled
disguised
disgust
disgusted
disgusting
disharmonious
disheartened
disheveled
dishonest
dishonorable
dishonored
disillusioned
disinclined

disingenuous
disinterested
dislocated
dislodged
disloyal
dismal
dismayed
dismissed
dismissive
disobedient
disobeyed
disorderly
disorganized
disoriented
disowned
disparaged
dispassionate
dispensable
dispirited
displaced
displeased
disposable
dispossessed
disputed
disquieted
disregarded
disrespected
disruptive
dissatisfied
dissected
dissed
dissident
dissipated
dissociated
distant
distorted
distracted

distraught
distressed
distrust
divided
divorced
dizziness (vertigo, spinning)
docile
dogged
dogmatic
doleful
domestic
domesticated
dominant
dominated
dominating
domineered
domineering
done
'don't understand'
doomed
duped
doormat
dorky
doted on
doting
double-crossed
doubted
doubtful
dowdy
down
down and out
down in the dumps
downcast
downhearted
downtrodden
drained
dramatic

drastic
drawn away
drawn back
drawn in
drawn toward
dread
dreaded
dreadful
dreamy
dreary
dried up
driven
droopy
dropped
drowning
drubbed
drummed
drunk
dry
dubious
dull
dulled
dumb
dumbfounded
dumped
dumped on
duped
dutiful
dwarfed
dynamic
dysfunctional
dysphonic

E

eager
early

earnest
earthy
eased
easy
easy-going
ebullient
eccentric
eclectic
eclipsed
economical
ecstatic
edgy
edified
edifying
educated
effaced
effective
effeminate
effervescent
effete
efficacious
efficient
effusive
egocentric
egotistic
egotistical
elastic
elated
elevated
elderly
electric
electromagnetic
electrified
elegant
elevated
eloquent
elusive

emancipated
emasculated
embarrassed
embittered
embracing
emerged
eminent
emotional
emotional boundaries
emotional stress
emotionless
emotionally bankrupt
emotionally bloated
emotionally-constipated
emotive
empathy
empowered
empty
empty of enmity
enraged
enabled
enamored
enchanted
enclosed
encompassed
encouraged
encroached-upon
encumbered
endangered
ending
endowed
endured
enduring
energetic
energized
enervated
engaged

engrossed
engulfed
enhanced
enigmatic
enjoyment
enlightened
enlivened
enmeshed
ennobled
enraged
enraptured
enriched
enslaved
entangled
enterprising
entertained
enthralled
enthusiastic
enticed
enticing
entitled
entombed
entranced
entrapped
entrenched
entrepreneurial
entrusted
envious
equality
erratic
energy
error
escape
escapism
estrangement
evasive
evicted

evil
eviscerated
exacerbated
exacerbating
examined
exasperated
exasperating
exasperation
excellent
excessive
excitable
excited
excluded
excoriated
exculpated
execrated
excused
exempt
exempted
exhausted
exhilarated
exiled
exigent
exonerated
exorcised
exotic
expansive
expectant
experienced
experimental
exploitative
exploited
explosive
exposed
expressive
expunged
extraordinary

extravagant
extreme
extricated
extroverted
exuberant
exultant

F

fabulous
facetious
factious
failure
faithfulness
faithful
faint
fainthearted
fair
faith
faithful
fake
fallen
fallible
fallow
false
falsely
falsely accused
faltering
family
famished
famous
fanatical
fanciful
fantabulous
fantasizing
fantastic
farcical

fascinated
fascinating
fascination
flashed
fashionable
fast
fastidious
fatalistic
fathered
fatherless
fatigued
fatuous
favored
fawned
fawned over
fawning
fazed
fear
feared
fearful
fearless
feckless
fed up
feeble
feeling
feisty
felicitous
feminine
fermenting
ferocious
fervent
fervor
festive
fettered
fickle
fidgety
fiendish

fierce
fiery
fighting
filthy
fine
finicky
finished
fired
firm
first
first-class
first-rate
fit
fixated
flabbergasted
flagellated
flaky
flamboyant
flammable
flappable
flat
flattered
flawed
fledgling
fleeced
flexible
flighty
flimflammed
flimsy
flip
flippant
flipped-out
flirtatious
flogged
floored
fluid
flummoxed

floundering
flourishing
flush
flustered
fluttering
focused
fogged in
focus (lack of)
foggy
foiled
followed
fond
foolhardy
foolish
forbearance
forbearing
forbidden
forced
forceful
foreign
fore-sighted
forgetful
forgettable
foggy
forgivable
forgiven
forgiving
forgotten
forlorn
formed
formidable
forsaken
fortified
fortunate
forward
foul
fouled

fouled-up
foundation
fractured
fragile
fragmented
frail
framed
frank
frantic
fraternal
fraternal loyalty
fraudulent
frazzled
freaked
freaked out
freakish
freaky
free
frenetic
frenzied
fresh
fret-filled
fretful
fretting
fried
friend out
friendless
friendly
frightened
frigid
frisky
frivolous
frolicsome
frowning
frugal
fruitful
frustrated

frustration
f-you
f--ked
fufilled
full
full of (feeling word)
full of life
full on
fuming
fun
functional
funky
fun-loving
funny
furious
fury
fussy
futile

G

gagged
gallant
galled
galvanized
game
garbled
garrulous
gather together
gauche
gaudy
gawky
gay
generous
genial
gentle
gentleness

genuine
ghastly
giddy
gilded
giving
glad
glamorized
glamorous
glee
gleeful
glib
gloomy
glorious
glowing
glum
gluttonous
goofed
goose bumpy
gnawing
goaded
gobsmacked
gobstruck
goober
good
good-humored
good-looking
good-natured
goofy
gorgeous
gory
gothic
graceful
gracious
graded
grand
grandiose
granted

grateful
gratified
grave
great
greedy
greeting
gregarious
grey
grief
grief-stricken
grieved
grieving
grim
groovy
gross
grossed-out
grotesque
grouchy
grounded
groveling
grown
grown-up
growth
grumpy
guarded
guided
guilt-free
guilt-tripped
guiltless
guilty
gullible
gushy
gutless
gutsy
gutted
gyped

H

haggard
haggled
hallowed
hammered
hampered
handicapped
hapless
happy
happy-go-lucky
harangued
harassed
hard
hardened
hard-headed
hard-hearted
hard-pressed
hard-working
hardy
harmless
harmonious
harnessed
harried
hassled
haste
hasty
hate
hate of God
hate of life
hate of self
hate of women
hated
hateful
hatred
haughty
haunted
hazy

headstrong
heady
healed
health abuse
health-conscious
healthy
heard
heartbroken
heartened
heartfelt
heartless
heartsick
heart-to-heart
hearty
heavy
heavy-hearted
heckled
heeded
held back
held dear
helped
helpful
helpless
henpecked
herded
heroic
hesitant
hideous
high
high-spirited
hilarious
hindered
hoaxed
holding
hollow
homely
homesick

homophobic
homosexual
honest
honorable
honored
hoodwinked
hopeful
hopeless
hormonal
horny
horrendous
horrible
horrific
horrified
horror
horror-stricken
hospitable
hostile
hot
hot to trot
hot-headed
hot-tempered
hounded
huge
humane
humble
humbled
humdrum
humiliated
humiliation
humility
humored
humorous
hung up
hung over
hungry
hunky dory

hunted
hurried
hurt
hustled
hyped-up
hyper
hyperactive
hyper-vigilant
hype
hypnotized
hypocritical
hysterical

I

I can't
I don't matter
idealistic
identify
idiosyncratic
idiotic
idle
idolized
ignoble
ignominious
ignorant
ignored
ill
ill at ease
ill-humored
ill-tempered
illicit
illuminated
imaginative
imbalanced
immaculate
immature

immobile
immobilized
immodest
immoral
immune
impractical
impressed
imprisoned
improve
improvise
impudent
impugned
impulsive
impure
in a huff
in a quandary
in a stew
in alignment
in control
in common
in despair
in doubt
in fear
in harmony
in love
in pain
in the dumps
in the way
in touch
in tune
inaccessible
inactive
inadequate
inane
inappropriate
inattentive
incapable

incapacitated
incensed
incongruence
incoherent
incommunicative
incompetent
incomplete
inconceivable
inconclusive
incongruent
inconsiderate
inconsistent
inconsolable
inconspicuous
incontinence
inconvenienced
inconvenient
incorrect
incorrigible
incredible
incredulous
inculcated
indebted
indecent
indecisive
indefinite
independent
indescribable
indestructible
indicted
indifferent
indignant
indirect
indiscreet
indoctrinated

indolent
indulgent
industrious
inebriated
ineffective
ineffectual
inefficient
inept
inert
inequality
inexplicable
infallible
infamous
infantile
infantized
infatuated
infected
inferior
infirm
inflamed
inflammatory
inflated
inflexible
influenced
influential
informed
infuriated
infused
ingenious
ingenuous
ingratiated
ingratiating
inhibited
inhospitable
inhumane
inimical
injured

injustices
innocent
innovative
inoculated
inquiring
inquisitive
insane
insatiable
inscrutable
insecure
insensitive
inside-out
insightful
insignificant
insincere
insistent
insolent
insouciant
inspired
instability
instilled
instructive
insufficient
insulted
insulting
insurgent
intact
integrities
intellectual
intelligent
intense
intent
interaction
interested
interesting
interfered with
interfering

interrelated
interrogated
interrupted
intimate
intimidated
intimidating
inoculated
intolerant
intoxicated
intrepid
intrigued
introspective
introverted
intruded upon
intrusive
inundated
intuitive
invalidated
invalidating
inventive
invigorated
invisible
invited
inviting
involved
invulnerable
irascible
irate
ire
irked
irrational
irreligious
irreproachable
irresistible
irresolute
irresponsible
irreverent

irritable
irritated
isolated
itchy

J

jaded
jangled
jaundiced
jaunty
jazzed
jealous
jealousy
jeared
jeopardized
jerked around
jilted
jinxed
jittery
jocular
jolly
jolted
jostled
jovial
joyful
joyless
joyous
jubilant
judged
judgmental
judicious
juggled
juiced
juiced up
jumbled

jumpy
junk
junked
junky
just
justice
justified

K

kicked around
kicked back
kindled
kind
kindhearted
kindly
kingly
kinky
knackered
knightly
knocked
knocked down
knocked out
knotted
knotted up
know-it-all
knowing
knowledgeable
known
kooky

L

labeled
labile
lascivious

lackadaisical
lacking
lackluster
laconic
lagging behind
laid-back
lambasted
lame
lamentful
lamenting
lampooned
languid
languishing
lashing out
late
laughable
laughed at
lavished
lax
lazy
led astray
leaned on
leaning
lecherous
lectured to
leery
left out
left behind
legitimate
let down
lethargic
letting go
level-headed
lewd
liable
liberal
liberated

licentious
lied about
lied to
life (suppression of)
lifeless
lifelike
lifted light
light-hearted
likeable
liked
liking
limerent
limited
limp
lionhearted
listened to
listening
litigious
lively
living together
loath
loathed
loathsome
logical
lonely
lonesome
longing
loopy
loose
loosed
lorded over
losing
loss
lost
loud
lousy
lovable

love
loved
loveless
lovely
loving
love-struck
low
low-spirited
lowly
lowness
loyal
lubrucious
luckless
lucky
ludicrous
luminous
lured
luring
lurking
lust
lustful
lusty
lying
lynched

M

made fun of
magical
magnificent
maimed
making love
maladjusted
malaise
maligned
malcontent
malleable

malevolent
malicious
malignant
maligned
malnourished
man handled
manageable
managed
managerial
mangled
maniacal
manic
manipulability
manipulated
manipulative
manly
marauding
marginalized
married
marshaled around
marvelous
masochistic
mass consciousness
masterful
materialistic
maternal
mature
maudlin
meager
mean
meanness
mechanical
medicated
mediocre
meditative
manic
meek

meeting
megalomaniacal
melancholic
melancholy
melded
mellow
melodramatic
menaced
menacing
merciful
mercy
merging
merry
mesmerized
messed around
messed with
messed up
messy
methodical
meticulous
micro-managed
miffed
mighty
militant
mind chatter
mindful
minimized
miraculous
mirthful
misanthropic
mischievous
misdiagnosed
miserable
misery
miserly
misgiving
misguided

misinformed
misinterpreted
misled
misrepresented
missed
missed out
missing out
mistaken
mistreated
mistrusted
mistrustful
misunderstanding
misunderstood
misused
mixed-up
mobilized
mocked
mocking
modern
modest
molded
molested
mollified
mollycoddled
monitored
monopolized
monstrous
moody
mopey
moping
moral
moralistic
morbid
mordant
moribund
moronic
morose

mortified
mothered
mothering
motherless
motherly
motivated
mournful
mouthy
moved
muddled
muffled
multi-directional
mummified
mushy
musical
mutuality
mutinied
mutinous
muzzled
mysterious
mystical
mystified

N

nagged
nailed
naive
naked
namby pamby
nameless
nannied
narcissistic
narrow-minded
nasty
natural
naughty

nauseated
neat
necessary
needed
needled
needy
negated
negative
negativity
neglected
negligent
nervous
nervy
nesting
nestled
nettled
neurotic
neutral
nice
nifty
niggardly
niggled
nihilistic
nit-picked
nit-picking
nit-picky
noble
noisy
nomadic
nonchalant
noncommittal
nonconforming
nonexistent
nonplused
normal
nosey
nostalgic

nothing
noticed
not good enough
not safe to
not worthy
not valued
nourished
nourishing
nudged
null
nullified
numb
numbed
nursed
nurturing
nuts
nutty

O

obedient
obeyed
objectified
obligated
obliged
obliging
obliterated
oblivious
obnoxious
obscene
obscured
obsequious
observant
observed
obsessed
obsessive
obstinate

obstructed
obvious
odd
off
off the hook
offended
offensive
officious
ogre-ish
okay
old
old-fashioned
omnipotent
on call
on display
on time
one-upped
open
open-minded
opinionated
opportunistic
opposed
opposition
oppositional
oppressed
optimistic
opulent
orderly
organized
ornery
orphaned
ostentatious
ostracized
ousted
out of balance
out of control
out of it

out of place
out of sorts
out of style
out of touch
out of tune
outdated
outdone
outgoing
outlandish
outnumbered
out-powered
outraged
outrageous
outranked
out-reasoned
outspoken
over
over-controlled
over-depended upon
over-done
over-protected
over-ruled
over-simplified
overanxious
overbearing
overcome
overdrawn
overestimated
overjoyed
overloaded
overlooked
overpowered
oversensitive
overwhelmed
overworked
overwrought
overzealous

owed
owing
owned
ownership
owning

P

pacified
paid off
pain
pained
painful
paired
paired-off
paired up
pampered
panic
panicked
panicky
paralyzed
paranoid
parasitic
pardoned
parsimonious
partial
passed by
passed off
passed over
passed up
passionate
passive
pastoral
paternal
pathetic
patient
patronized

payback
peaceful
peachy
peckish
peculiar
pedantic
pedestalized
pedestrian
peeved
peevish
pell-mell
penetrable
penetrated
pensive
peppy
percieved
perceptive
peremptory
perfect
perfectionist
perilous
peripheral
perky
permanent
permeable
perplexed
persecuted
persevering
persistent
persnickety
perspicuous
persuaded
persuasive
pert
pertinacious
pertinent
perturbed

perverted
pervious
pessimistic
pestered
petered out
petrified
petty
petulant
philanthropic
phlegmatic
phony
picked apart
picked on
pierced
pigeon holed
pillaged
pillaging
pious
pissed
pissed off
pissy
piteous
pitied
pitiful
pitiless
pity
pixilated
placated
placid
plagued
plain
plaintive
painless
played with
playful
pleading
pleasant

pleased
pleasure
pliable
pliant
plumbed
plundered
plundering
plunging
plush
poised
poisoned
polite
polluted
pompous
pooped
poor
popular
porous
portentous
positive
possessed
possession less
possessive
potent
pouty
powerful
powerless
practical
praised
pragmatic
preached to
precarious
precious
precluded
precocious
preoccupied
prepared

preppy
pressed
pressured
presumptuous
pretentious
pretty
prayed upon
pride
prim
primal
primary
pristine
private
privileged
privy
prized
proactive
probationary
probationer
probed
prodigal
prodigious
productive
profane
professional
progressing
progressive
progress-minded
promiscuous
promised
promoted
promotional
prone to
propagandistic
propagandized
propelled
proper

prosaic
prosecuted
protecting
proud
punched
punished
puny
pure
purged
purposeful
pursuant
pursued
pushed
pushed ahead
pushed away
pushed back
provoked
prudish
psyched
psychopathic
psychotic
puerile
puffed up
pulled
pulled ahead
pulled apart
pulled away
pulled back
pulled down
pulled forward
pulled in
pulverized
pummeled
pumped
pumped up
punctual
punch drunk

punched
punished
punishment
puny
pure
purged
purplish
purposeful
pursuant
pursued
pushed
pushed back
pushed forward
pushed in
pushy
pusilianimous
put away
put down
put out
put upon
put down
puzzled
psychedelic

Q

quaint
quaking
qualified
qualmish
quandary
quarantined
quarrelsome
quashed
questioned
questioning

quick
quiescent
quiet
quietened
quirky
quivery
quixotic
quizzed
quizzical

R

radiant
radical
rage
rambunctious
ransacked
rancid
rancorous
rapacious
raped
rapt
rapture
rapturous
rare
rash
rated
rational
rattled
raunchy
ravenous
ravished
reachable
reactionary
reactive
ready

real
realistic
reamed
reamed out
reasonable
reassured
rebellious
reborn
rebounding
rebuffed
rebuked
recalcitrant
receptive
reciprocal
reckless
recovered
recruited
redeemed
red-hot
re-energized
re-enforced
reduced
refectory
reference
refined
reflective
refreshed
refueled
regimented
regressing
regressive
regret
regretful
rejectable
relaxed
relaxation
released
releasing
reliable
reliant
relieved
relief
religious
religiosity
reluctant
remedied
reminiscent
remiss
remorse
remorseful
remorseless
remote
removed
renewed
replaced
replenished
repelled
reprehensible
repressed
reprimanded
reproached
reproved
repugnant
repulsed
repulsive
rescued
resented
resentful
resentment
reserved
resigned
resilient
resistant
respected

respectful
responsible
responsive
rested
restful
restive
restless
restrained
restricted
resurrection
retaliated
retaliated against
retaliatory
retarded
reticent
retired
reunited
revenge
reviled
revitalized
revisited
revived
revolted
revolting
revolutionary
rewarded
rich
ridden
ridiculed
ridiculous
riding high
right
righteous
rigid
rigorous
riled
risky

riveted
robbed
robotic
robust
romantic
rotten
rough
rowdy
rubbery
rubricated
rude
rueful
ruffled
ruined
ruled
run down
run out
run over
running away
rushed
rut
ruthless

S

sabotaged
sacrificed
sacrificial
sacrilegious
sad
sadistic
safe
sagacious
sage
salacious
sanctified
sanctifying

sanctimonious
sanctioned
sane
sanguine
sapient
sarcastic
sardonic
sassy
sated
satiated
satisfied
saucy
saved
savvy
scandalized
scandalous
scapegoat
scared
scarred
scathed
scattered
scheming
scientific
scintillated
scurrilous
scoffed at
scolded
scorn
scorned
scornful
screwed
screwed over
screwed up
scrutinized
sealed out
scaled in
sealed off

sealed up
seared
secondary
second-class
second-guessed
second-rate
secure
sedate
seduced
seductive
seeing (fear of)
seething
seized
selected
selective
self-absorbed
self-acceptance
self-acceptant
self-aggradizing
self-assured
self-blame
self-centered
self-confident
self-conscious
self-denial
self-doubt
self-depracating
self-depreciating
self-destructive
self-disciplined
self-effacing
self-esteem (low)
self-expressed
self-flagellating
self-forgiving
self-hate
self-hating

self-hatred
self-indulgent
self-limitation
self-loathing
self-love
self-pitying
self-pleasing
self-rejection
self-reliant
self-righteous
self-sacrificing
self-serving
self-understanding
selfish
selfless
senile
sensational
sensible
sensing
sensitive
sensual
sensuous
sentenced
sentimental
separated
serene
serendipitous
serious
servile
set
set up
settled
settling
scores
sexy
shadowed
shaken

shaky
shallow
shamed
shameful
shaped
sharing
sharp
shattered
sheepish
sheltered
shielded
shocked
shook-up
shortchanged
shot-down
shouted at
shredded
shrewd
shrunk
shrunken
shunned
shut out
shut down
shy
sick
sick at heart
sickened
side-lined
significant
silenced
silent
silly
simple
simplified
sincere
sinful
single

singled-out
sinking
skanky
skeptical
skilled
skillful
skipped
skittish
slack
slain
slandered
slaughtered
sleazy
sleepy
slap happy
slave
sledged
slighted
sloppy
sloshed
slothful
slovenly
slow
slugged
sluggish
slutty
small
smarmy
smart
smart-alecky
smart assy
smacked
smacked down
smashed
smitten
smooth
smothered

smudged
smug
snapped at
snarky
snarled at
sneaky
snobbish
snobby
snoopy
snowed
snubbed
snuggled
soaring
sociable
social
sodden
soft
soft-hearted
sold
sold-out
solemn
solid
solitary
somber
'something is wrong with me'
soothed
sophisticated
sophomoric
sorcery
sordid
sore
sorrow
sorrowful
sorry
sound
sour
soured

spared
sparkling
spartan
spastic
special
speechless
spellbound
spent
spineless
spinning wheels (frustrated)
spirited
spiritless
spiteful
splendid
splendiferous
spoiled
spontaneous
spooked
spunky
squandered
squashed
squeamish
squeezed
squelched
stable
stained
stale
stagnation
stalked
startled
starved
static
steamed-up
stepped-on
stepped-over
stereotyped
sterile

stern
stewing
stiff
stifled
stigmatized
still
stilted
stimulated
stingy
stirred
stodgy
stoic
stolid
stomped on
stoned
stonewalled
stout
stout-hearted
straight-laced
strained
stranded
strange
strangled
strengthened
stressed (physical/emotion)
stretched
stricken
strict
stroked
strong
strong-armed
strong-willed
struck
struck down
stubborn
stuck-up
studious

stuffed
stumped
stunned
stunning
stunted
stupefied
stupid
stylish
suave
subdued
subjugated
submissive
subordinate
subordinated
subservient
subtle
subversive
successful
sucked up to
suckered
suffering
suffocated
suicidal
sulky
sullen
sullied
sunk
sunny
super
superb
supercilious
superficial
superior
superseded
superstitious
supported
supportive

suppressed
sure
surly
surpassed
surprised
surreal
surrendered
surveyed
survival
susceptible
suspended
suspending
suspicious
strong
struggle
stubborn
stuck
success (fear of)
swallowed emotions
swamped
sweet
swell
swindled
switched on
sycophantic
symmetrical
sympathetic
sympathy

T

taciturn
telling
terrified
threatened
tired
touchy

trapped
troubled
tactless
taker
talk too much
temperamental
tempted
tenderness
tentativeness
tenuousness
tense
tender
tension
terrible
terror/terrified
tepid
thankful
thankfulness
thin-skinned
thoughtfulness
thoughtless
thrilled
threatened
thwarted
ticked-off
timid
tired
tormented
touched
toxicity
traitor
trauma
trust
trembling
tribulation
troubled
truthful

turmoil (in)
tranquil
trusting
turned off
two-faced
tyrannical

U

ugly
unable
unable to express self
unacceptable
unaware
unbearable
unbelief
uncertain
uncharitable
unclear
uncomfortable
uncompromising
unconcerned
unconscious
uncontrollable
undecided
undesirable
undeserving
undisciplined
uneasy
unfulfilled
used
useless
upbeat
uptight
unfair
unfeeling

unfit
unforgiveable
unforgivingness
unfriendly
unfulfilled
ungrateful
ungrounded
unhappy
unimportant
unjust
unimportant
unkind
unknown
unlovable
unloved
unloving
unlucky
unmerciful
unmindful
unnerved
unnoticed
unorganized
unpleasant
unpopular
unprepared
unproductive
unprotected
unqualified
unreasonable
unreceptive
unrelenting
unreliable
unrepentant
unresolved (of anything)
unsatisfied needs
unsettled
unstable

unsuccessful
unsteady
unsupported
unsure (of self)
unthankful
untidy
untrusting
untrustworthy
untruthful
unwanted
unwelcome
unwilling (to change)
unwise
unworthy
unyielding
upset
uptight
used
useless
utilized

V

victimized
violated
vulnerable
vulnerability
vague
vain
vehemence
vengeful
versed
vexed
vicious
victim (like a)
vindictive
violated

violence (self)
violent
vitality
vivaciousness
void
vulgar
vow

W

wallowing
warm
wasted
wary
wavering
weak
weak-minded
wide-awake
weary
weepy
what is the use?
what is wrong with me?
will
why me?
wicked
willful
wishy-washy
wisdom (fear of)
wistfulness
withdrawn
withholding
woeful
worried
worry
worthless
wounded

wonderful
wretched
wrong (always)

Y

yearning

Z

zany
zestful
zippy

POSITIVE and UPLIFTING WORDS

Abundance
Awareness
Artistic creativity
Bounciness
Cheerfulness
Concern
Confidence
Constructiveness
Courage
Creativity
Drama
Elfishness playfulness
Enlightenment
Enthusiasm
Entertainment
Exhilaration
Facetious-joking or jesting
Forgive
Freedom

Gentleness
Gleefulness
Goofy playfulness
Happiness
Hope
Humor
Imagination
Joy
Kindness
Laughter
Love
Mercy
Mysterious
Perseverance
Playfulness
Poise
Relaxation
Self-control
Self-esteem
Self-preservation
Silliness playfulness
Strength
Supportiveness
Surprised wonder
Worthiness
Ticklish
Thoughtfulness
Trust
Vitality
Wonder

CHAPTER 6

The Human Brain

Areas of the Human Brain

The human brain and the nervous system are extremely important in the way the body functions and in the way that we integrate into our environment. For this reason it is important that we know the basic areas and functions of the brain and nervous system. Blockages of these areas can create a multitude of symptoms that can be extremely bothersome to the patient until they are cleared. If you find a blockage in the brain, be patient and go through these areas until you have cleared them all. The following are important areas of the brain and what function they serve.

AREAS OF THE BRAIN

Commissure

1. A line or a place at which two things are joined.

2. A tract of nerve fibers in the spinal cord or brain that pass from one side to the other

3. The point, angle, or surface where two parts, such as the eyelids, lips, or cardiac valves, join or connect.

Brain commissures

The brain commissures are the bands of fibers which connect the parts of the two cerebral hemispheres. These commissures include the corpus callosum (the largest commissure), a rostral commissure (which is part of the paleo-pallium), and the fornical commissure (which is related to the archipallium), the caudal col-licular commissure (which connects the caudal colliculi--corpora quadrigemina). This is also known as the cerebral commissure.

Hippocampus Commissure

The Hippocampus is a curved elevation of the floor of the inferior portion of the lateral ven-tricle of the human brain. It is made up of gray substance and covered by a layer of white fibers (the alveus), and it functions as a very important component of the limbic system, the portion of the brain that controls learning and

of memory processing. Its efferent projections
make up the fornix of the cerebrum. This portion of the brain is also called Ammon's horn
or the hippocampus major

Anterior Commissure

The anteror commissure is a collection of nerve
fibers which cross the midline of the spinal
cord. It acts to transmit information to or
from the opposite side of the brain.

Sylvian Fissure

The Sylvian fissure extends laterally between
the temporal and the frontal lobes of the brain.
They then turn posteriorly and can be found
between the temporal and parietal lobes. This
is also called the fissure of Sylvius, or the
lateral cerebral sulcus.

Corpus Collosum

The corpus collosum is an arched mass of
white matter that is found in the depths
of the longitudinal fissure. It is composed
of transverse fibers and is responsible
for connecting the right and left cerebral
hemispheres.

Habenular Commissure

This part of the brain creates the intricate
connection between the right and left

habenular nuclei.

Posterior Commissure

The Posterior Commissure is a large fiber bundle which crosses from one side of the cerebrum to the other dorsal to where the aqueduct opens up into the third ventricle.

Cerebellum

The cerebellum is a trilobed structure within the brain. It lies posterior to the pons and medulla oblongata and it is inferior to the occipital lobes. The cerebellum is responsible for the regulation and coordination of complex voluntary movement in the body and for the maintenance of posture and balance.

Thalamus

The thalamus is one of a pair of large oval structures made of gray matter and forming most of the lateral walls of the third ventricle of the brain and part of the diencephalon. This part of the brain relays sensory information, excluding smell, to the cortex. It is composed mainly of gray substance and it translates impulses from various receptors into crude sensations including pain, temperature, and touch. The thalamus also aids in associating sensory impulses with pleasant and unpleasant feelings, in the arousal mechanisms of the body, and in the mechanisms that produce complex reflex movements.

Superior and Inferior Colliculus midbrain colliculus

There are four total colliculi in the midbrain. These include two caudal (inferior) and two rostral (superior) and they contain the visual and auditory reflex centers. These are also called the corpora quadrigemina.

Collicular Commissures

Medial View

Relating to, situated in, or extending toward the middle; median.

Coronal View

1. Relating to a corona, especially of the head.

2.Relating to, or having the direction of the coronal suture or of the plane dividing the body into front and back portions.

Right Hemisphere

Speech – Written

Information Processing

Inferior

The lateral region of the cerebrum. It is

located below the lateral fissure. This part of
the brain contains the center for smell, some
areas having to do with memory and learning,
as well as a region having to do with choice
and thoughts of expression.

Ventral Pathway

This relates to either the anteror or the bottom
in regards to brain orientation.

Primary Visual Cortex

The primary visual cortex is the specific area of
the occipital lobe that is primarily dealing with
vision. It is the part of the cerebral corex that
deals with images relayed to the brain by the
visual sructures.

Occipital Lobe

The occipital lobe is the most posterior part
of the brain, forming a small part of the
dorsolateral surface of the cerebral hemisphere
surface.

Porsal(dorsal) Pathway Posterior Parietal Cortex

This is the upper middle portion of the cerebral
hemisphere. It is located between the frontal
and the occipital lobes of the brain. It is above
the temporal lobe

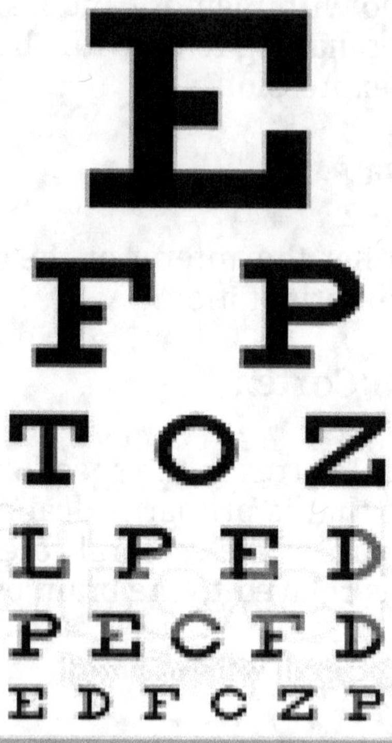

E Z V U R (10)

D U N R P (12.5)

V E N U H (16)

D N R U P (20)

Z H E D N (25)

R P U F D (32)

H N P V F (40)

E Z F D V (50)

The Body and Nutrition

Food and Nutritients

It is important to check for food allergies and sensitivities. Food allergies and sensitivities can manifest in all sorts of ways in the body and can be very easily overlooked. Nutritional deficiencies can also play a part. So it is extremely important that food and nutrition within the body and in a patient's life be addressed. For instance, many people have problems with eggs and they might not even know it.

The following is a list of foods you can check for. I have split them into groups and organized them by the metals they contain.

Possible Allergens and their Descriptions

EGGS

Eggs are typically an oval or round object that is laid by a female bird, reptile, fish, or invertebrate. And they usually contain a developing embryo. The eggs of birds are enclosed in a chalky shell, while those of reptiles surrounded by a more leathery membrane. Eggs are one of the most common causes of allergies in children. Many people will outgrow the allergy before adolescence, but not all.

Symptoms of an egg allergy can be anywhere from mild reactions to a severe allergic reaction (anaphylaxis). The most common symptoms found in an egg allergy are reactions associated with the skin. Other symptoms may include runny nose and itchy and watery eyes (similar to hay fever), cramps, nausea or vomiting. The best way to manage an egg allergy is by elimination, avoiding all food containing egg or egg products. A study published in the American Journal of Clinical Nutrition has been sited to say that the men who ate seven eggs a week or more were 23 percent more likely to have died during the 20-year period. However, men with diabetes who ate any eggs at all raised their risk of death during the same amount of time.

Eggs are rich in cholesterol, which in high amounts can clog arteries and raise the risk of heart attack and stroke. To be fair, men who ate the most eggs also were older, fatter, ate more vegetables but less breakfast cereal, and were more likely to drink alcohol, smoke and less likely to exercise — all factors that can affect the risk of heart attack and death.

SOY PROTEIN

This is a protein that is pulled from dehulled and defatted soybeans. It can be found in a great number of products, including pet food and salad dressing. It frequently shows up as an allergen often, especially in women.

DNA

Stands for deoxyribose nucleic acid. It is the instructions for the building of our bodies and how they should function. These instructions are relayed by the order in which 4 amino acids line up and create a double helix formation. They can go hay-wire (or get better) from random mutations.

GENETICALLY MODIFIED ORGANISMS (GMO'S)

All foods are modified though their DNA, one way or the other. However, the term 'GMO' refers to foods that are modified by directly inserting a gene into a plant's genome without the act of cross-breeding or irradiating plants.

CALCIUM CASEINATE

This protein is produces from adding an alkali to casein, such as in dry milk. It can be found in a variety of products, including coffee creamers, instant soups, and protein supplements for body-builders.

FRUCTOSE

Fructose is a type of sugar and it is a monosacharide. It results from your body breaking down more complex sugars. Fructorse can be found in fruits and sweet vegetables as well as high fructose corn syrup. Honey is almost completely made up of fructose and makes things sweet.

MAGNESIUM PHOSPHATE

This chemical is the result of combining salts of magnesium and phosphate. Variations of the results are often used as laxatives and antacids. It comes in the following three types:

Magnesium phosphate monobasic $(Mg(H_2PO_4)_2)$
Magnesium phosphate dibasic $(MgHPO_4)$
Magnesium phosphate tribasic $(Mg_3(PO_4)_2)$

CASEIN

Casein comes from the salt of calcium. It is found in many dairy products and is also used in the making of plastics, paints, and the like.

POTASSIUM BICARBONATE

Potassium bicarbonate is a slightly alkaline, salty substance that comes from combining potassium and carbon dioxide. It is used to regulate the acidity of many products, including soil. It can be extracted straight from the ground, but you will most commonly find it in soda water, supplements for people low on potassium, and as a leavener in baked goods.

GUAR GUM

Guar gum is a water soluble fiber. It is sometimes also called guaran. It can be found in a variety of foods as an additive that improves texture and prolongs a products usable life. Some industries use it for making products thicker and better stabilized. It is produced from guar beans, and can be used in laxatives as well as in products designed to make you feel full for longer.

DIPOTASSIUM PHOSPHATE

Other names for dipotassium phosphate include phosphoric acid, dipotassium salt, dipotassium hydrogen orthophosphate, potassium phosphate, and dibasic. It comes from combining phosphorus and potassium to create a highly-water soluble salt. Food producers add it to foods in order to increase the potassium and phosphate levels and make products easier to cook with.

MONOGLYCERIDE

A monoglyceride is formed when a glycerol and a fatty acid hook up through an ester bond. Food production companies love monoglycerides because they keep oil and water from separating in products like margarine, ice cream, and baked goods. They also prevent bread from going stale right away.

SUCRALOSE

Sucralose is fake sugar put in diet foods. Most of it doesn't break down in the body after you eat it. You make it by chlorinating sucrose a couple times.

IRON (III) PHOSPHATE

Iron phosphate is also called ferric orthophosphate, or ferric phosphate, $FePO_4$. It is produced by combining phosperous, iron and oxygen. Food companies use it to fortify breads, pasta, milks, and some other beverages. It can be found naturally in water and other types of foods.

TOCOPHEROL (VITAMIN E)

Vitamin E can be found in eight different forms, and each one is used by the body in slightly different ways. It can be found in cosmetics, You can also get it orally from peanut butter, goat's milk, nuts, vegetable oil, and a bunch of other oily things.

ZINC SULFATE

Zinc sulfate is a colorless crystaline chemical that disolves easily in water. It comes from adding aqueous sulferic acid to zinc. You can also add zinc to copper II sulfate. It gets added to supplements to combat zinc deficiencies.

PANTOTHENIC ACID

Pantothenic Acid is the formal name for B5. It can be found in meats and a variety of other foods.

CALCIUM (AS 'ALBION' CALCIUM AMINO ACID CHELATE)

Calcium is an element and an essential nutrient that can be found in milk, brocolli and a variety of other foods. It acts to strengthen your bones and can be added to foods to make them more alkaline, and to change the texture of everything.

MANGANESE (II) SULFATE

Manganese (II) sulfate is a solid, pale pink compound which tends to easily move to its liquid form. You can get it in the form of Epsom salt. It can be used to settle your stomach, soothe tired muscles when you add it to a bath, and fertilize plants. Food processors add it to flour, cheese, and candy. Brewers use it to make beer.

PYRIDOXINE

Pyridoxine is a form of Vitamin B6. It an be

found in fruit, vegetables and grains, and it is used in the body to make amino acids and lipids. It can be prescribed by a doctor as an antidote to a certain type of anemia and metabolic disorders. It gets added to breads and cereals sometimes as well.

THIAMIN MONONITRATE

About half of the body stores of thiamin are found in skeletal muscles, with the remainder dispersed throughout the heart, liver, kidneys, and nervous tissues, including the brain. Thiamine and B12 are the only vitamins whose deficiencies have proven causes of neurologic disease. It takes only three weeks of a total dietary lack of thiamin to see the first signs of deficiency.

Thiamin's enzyme helper is "thiamin pyrophosphate," (TPP) needed to break down glucose, fats and carbohydrates vital for energy production. Thiamin promotes a normal appetite; aids in digestion; helps fight off motion sickness; keeps the nervous system, muscles and heart functioning normally; improves mental attitude; and has proven effective in the treatment of lead toxicity. Studies show that increased thiamin dosage stimulates neutrophil chemotaxis, an attraction of cells into an area of inflammation, thereby speeding the healing process.

Thiamin deficiency occurs as a result of many factors, including crash dieting, alcohol abuse, liver disfunction, kidney dialysis, and sustained periods of IV nutrients. Also at risk are those who consume a lot of sweets, soft drinks, and highly processed foods. Alcohol not only blocks thiamin assimilation but injures the small intestine, making nutrient absorption in general very difficult. Similarily, tea, coffee (both caffeinated and decaffeinated), and the chewing of betelnuts or tea leaves deplete thiamine, as do some medications and cigarette smoke. The heating of food and processing can destroy this fragile vitamin. However, microwave cooking does not seem to increase vitamin loss, despite claims to the contrary. In addition, thiamin is poorly absorbed when there is a folacin or protein deficiency. Clinically similar to thiamin deficiency is a form of polyneuropathy, a disease involving several nerves, which does not respond to thiamin thereapy. It usually occurs in uncontrolled or long-continued forms of diabetes. A deficiency can also masquerade as senility, but supplementation does not affect mental processes if thiamin deficiency is not the cause. A thiamin deficiency also produces Warnicke-Korsakoff syndrome, sometimes called "cerebral beriberi," a disorder of the central nervous system.

Deficiencies can be classified within three reasons:

1) the body requires more than normal as in cases of hyperthyroidism, pregnancy, lactation, and fever
2) there is impaired absorption caused by prolonged diarrhea or lack of necessary enzymes, for example
3) there is impaired utilization brought on by severe liver impairment or other disorders.

Other names for thiamin include: Vitamin B1,
formerly Vitamin F, aneurin, polyneuramin,
oryzamin, antineuritio factor/vitamin,
antuberiberi factor/vitamin.

Its forms are: thiamine/B1 disulfide, thiamine
hydrochloride, thiamine mononitrate, thiamine
phosphoric acid ester chloride, thiamine
phosphoric acid ester phosphate salt, thiamine
1, 5-salt, Vitamin B1 propyl disulfide, thiamine
triphosphoric acid ester, thiamine
triphosphoric acid salt, thiamine/Vitamin B1 O,
S diacetate, thiamin pyrophosphate.

Inhibitors are: cooking, fevers,
hyperthyroidism, liver and digestion
deterioration, tannins or tannic acid,
chlorogenic acid in coffee, baking soda,
estrogen, antacids and barbiturates, and a
decreased availability of Vitamin B6 and B12.
Helpers are: B Complex vitamins, Vitamins B2,
B3, Bc, C, E, manganese, and sulfur.

Deficiency symptoms include: brain
deterioration, decreased memory, depression,
emotional agitation and deterioration,
decreased vision, inflammation of the optic
nerve, CNS and reflex deterioration, increased
pyruvic acid in the blood, tingling or burning
of feet, decreased sense of touch, fatigue,
decreased appetite and digestion, constipation,
decreased immunity, decreased protein
synthesis, abdominal and chest pains, cardiac
deterioration, decreased blood pressure,
varicose veins, bluish skin color, labored
breathing, tender leg muscles, decreased
resistance to cancers. Early signs include

fatigue, irritability, sensitivity to noise,
memory loss, inability to concentrate, fatigue,
sleep disturbances, precordial pain (area above
the heart), appetite loss, abdominal discomfort,
and constipation. Symptoms of moderate
deficiency include fatigue, apathy, nausea,
irritability, depression, slow wound healing,
loss of appetite, indigestion, constipation.
Other symptoms attributed to a thiamin
deficiency include: irregular heart beat,
shortness of breath, low blood pressure, chest
and abdominal pain, kidney failure, heart
failure, and death. Thiamin has proven to
correct all these symptoms -- with the
exception of the last one. Toxicity symptoms
include: muscle tremors, fluid accumulation,
skin inflammations, nervousness, heart
palpitations, allergies, altered thyroid and
insulin production, and too much decreases
Vitamin B6.

Vitamin B1 O,S-diacetate is a lipid-soluble
form of thiamin. Other names include:
thiamine O,S-diacetate, acetiamine,
Thianeuron.

Vitamin B1 disulfide is a specific form of
Vitamin B1.

Vitamin B1 hydrochloride is a special form of
Vitamin B1. Other names include: thiamin
hydrochloride, thiamin chloride hydrochloride,
aneurine hydrochloride, thiaminium chloride
hydrochloride, Bedome, Begiolan, Benerva,
Bequin, Berin, Betabion hydrochloride, Betalin
S, Betaxin, Bethiazine, Bevitex, Bewon, Biuno,
Bivatin, Bivita, Clotiamina, Metabolin,
Thiadoxine, Thiavit, Tiamidon, Tiaminal,

Vitaneuron.

Vitamin B1 mononitrate is a special form of
Vitamin B1. Other names include: aneurine
mononitrate, Betabion mononitrate.

Vitamin B1 Phosphoric acid ester chloride is a
special form of Vitamin B1. Other names
include: thiamin phosphoric acid ester
chloride, thiamin orthophosphate ester
chloride.

Vitamin B1 phosphoric acid ester salt is a
special form of Vitamin B1. Other names
include: thiamin monophosphate ester
phosphoric acid salt, Umbeon.

Vitamin B1 propyl disulfide is a lipid–form of
vitamin B1. Other names include: thiamin
propyl disulfide, DTPT, TPD, Prosultiamine,
Alinamin, Aneurimec, AusovitB1. Betatron,
Binova, Ditiovit, Liponeurina, Marineurina,
Orobetina, Proneurin, Sintotiamina, Tipidi.

Vitamin B1 1,5–salt is a form of Vitamin B1.
Other names include: thiamin 1,5–salt,
aneurin–1,5 salt; thiamin chloride
naphthalene–1,5–disulfonic acid salt.

Vitamin B1 triphosphoric acid ester is a special
form of Vitamin B1. Other names include:
thiamin triphosphoric acid ester, thiamin
triphosphate ester.

Vitamin B1 triphosphoric acid salt is a special
form of B1. Other names include: thiamin
triphosphoric acid salt, thiamin triphosphate
salt.

BIOTIN

Biotin is also known as vitamin H or B7. It is a water-soluble B-complex vitamin. Biotin is used in the metabolism and break down of fatty acids as well as leucine. It is also used in the process of gluconeogenesis. Biotin plays a large part in cell growth, in the synthesis of fatty acids, and in the breakdown of fats and amino acids. Biotin plays a role in the Citric acid cycle (the process in which biochemical energy is created during aerobic respiration). Biotin plays a part in many metabolic reactions in the body, and it helps to transfer carbon dioxide into the cell. Biotin is helpful in maintaining a steady blood sugar level. Biotin may be used to strengthen the hair and the nails and can be found in many cosmetic and products for the hair and skin.

A deficiency of Biotin is an extremely rare occurence, because the bacteria in your gut actually produces in excess of the body's daily requirement. For this reason, many institutions dealing with health requirements do not prescribe a recommended daily intake.

Biotin can be found in a variety of foods. Most often being found at low concentrations within food sources. There are very few foods which contain biotin in large amounts. These foods include royal jelly and brewer's yeast. The most important natural sources of biotin occuring naturally are in milk, liver, egg (egg yolk), and some vegetables.

It is of note that individuals with type 2 diabetes will often be found to have low levels of biotin. Biotin appears to be involved in the synthesis and release of insulin. Early studies in both animals and people show that biotin can help to improve blood glucose control in those with diabetes, particularly type 2 diabetes.[5] Specifically, biotin doses in excess of nutritional requirements lower postprandial glucose and improve glucose tolerance.[2]

A deficiency in Biotin is relatively mild, and may be dealt with through supplementation. A deficiency can be caused by excessive consumption of raw egg whites, which contain high levels of the protein avidin. Avidin strongly binds biotin limiting its levels in the body. Avidin can be deactivated by cooking, while the biotin remains intact.

VITAMIN K (PHYTONADIONE)

Vitamin K is part of a group of lipophilic, hydrophobic vitamins. These vitamins are needed for modification of certain proteins which play a great part in blood coagulation.

Vitamin K2 (menaquinone, menatetrenone) is produced by bacteria in the intestines, and deficiency of this vitamin is extremely rare unless there has been damage to the intestines, or there is a problem with absorbtion that prevent it from entrering the system. Blood coagulation: (prothrombin (factor II), factors VII, IX, X, protein C, protein S and protein Z). [3]

* Bone metabolism: osteocalcin, also called bone Gla-protein (BGP), and matrix gla protein

(MGP).[4]
* Vascular biology.[5]

Vitamin K can be found mostly in leafy green vegetables. The dark leafy ones are the most common to have high levels of Vitamin K. These include spinach and kale; Brassica, e.g. cabbage, cauliflower, broccoli, and brussels sprouts. Vitamin K is also found in some fruit such as avocado and kiwifruit.

Prescription drugs such as Warfarin and other coumarin drugs can actually block the action of the Vitamin K epoxide reductase.[30] This results in decreased amounts of Vitamin K and Vitamin K hydroquinone in the tissues. It creates a situation in which the carboxylation reaction catalyzed by the glutamyl carboxylase is inefficient.

GLA-PROTEINS

Currently, the following human Gla-containing proteins have been characterized primarily: the blood coagulation factors II (prothrombin), VII, IX, and X, the anticoagulant proteins C and S, and the Factor X-targeting protein Z. The bone Gla-protein osteocalcin, the calcification inhibiting matrix gla protein (MGP), the cell growth regulating growth arrest specific gene 6 protein, (Gas6), and the four transmembrane Gla proteins (TMGPs) the function of which is at present unknown. Gas6 can act as a growth factor which activates the Axl receptor tyrosine kinase and stimulates cell proliferation or prevents apoptosis in some cells. In all cases in which their function was known, the presence of the Gla-residues in these proteins turned out to be essential for functional activity.

Gla-proteins can be found in a wide variety of vertebrates: mammals, birds, reptiles, and fish. The venom of a number of Australian snakes acts by activating the Gla- proteins and the human blood clotting system.

MAGNESIUM CARBONATE

Magnesium carbonate, $MgCO_3$, is a white solid that occurs in nature as a mineral.

Magnesite and dolomite minerals are used to produce magnesium metal and basic refractory bricks. $MgCO_3$ is also used in flooring, fireproofing, fire extinguishing compositions, cosmetics, dusting powder, and toothpaste. It can also be used as filler material, smoke suppressant in plastics, a reinforcing agent in neoprene rubber, a drying agent, a laxative to loosen the bowels, and a factor in color retention in foods. It can also be used as an antacid in high purity forms as well as being used as an additive in table salt to keep it a free flowing texture.

Magnesium carbonate or E504, AKA 'chalk', is used most frequently as a drying agent for hands in rock climbing, gymnastics, and weight lifting.

Magnesium carbonate can also be used in taxidermy (preserving animals) for whitening skulls. It can be combined with hydrogen peroxide which creates a paste. That paste is then spread on the skull to produce a white finish.

Magnesium Carbonate Hydroxide is used in the production of face mask. It has mild astringent properties and helps to smooth and soften the skin. It is recommended for use on normal to dry skins.

CYANOCOBALAMIN

Cyanocolbalamin is a member of the B12 family. This can not be found naturally and therefor must be made in a lab. After it is produced, it can be used to supplement foods with B12. It breaks down into metabolites that your body recognizes and uses as if it were B12.

CARAMEL COLORING

Carmel Coloring is exactly what it sounds like. It is naturally occuring and can be added to foods to make them a beige color.

IRON

Iron is a trace mineral and it is required for red blood cell formation and adequate formation of hemoglobin. (Hemoglobin is a protein that carries oxygen in the blood and myoglobin, a similar protein that carries oxygen in the muscle tissue.) Iron plays an important part in many biochemical pathways and enzyme systems within the body. These include those involved with energy metabolism, neurotransmitter production (serotonin and dopamine), collagen formation and immune system function. Iron requirements are at their highest in normally menstruating women. Supplemental iron is rarely needed in young children, adult men and elderly women. Any supplementation in these groups should be preceded with a consult of a physician. There are many good food sources of iron. These include liver and other organ meats, red meat like beef, beans and peas. The form of iron found in meats is called heme iron and is much more absorbable than the type of iron (non-heme) found in plants. The non-heme iron found in beans and peas can be made more absorbable by eating foods rich in vitamin C such as citrus fruit or tomatoes. Iron supplements may help but they are NOT recommended for everybody. Chronically high intakes of iron can lead to the accumulation of iron in tissues such as the heart and liver, which can lead to toxic damage and increased risk for disease. Another condition called hemochromatosis (found primarily in middle-aged men) can lead to excessive iron absorption and accumulation of toxic iron levels in the heart, liver, spleen, and pancreas.

HIGH-FIBER FOODS

Fiber is a product that has the ability to move quickly and easily through the digestive tract. It helps with the function of the digestive tract and can reduce the risk of heart disease and diabetes. Current recommended fiber intake levels are labeled as 21 to 25 grams a day for women, and 30 to 38 grams a day for men.

COCHINEAL (DACTYLOPIUS COCCUS)

Cochineal is a bug from Mexico and is often crushed up and used to create the red color of certain foods.

CARRANGEENAN

Carrangeenan is actually just a fancy word for seaweed. It is used in certain foods such as ice cream, pudding, and other dairy products, to thicken them. According to Jacobson, it is extracted from red seaweed that's plentiful on the Irish coast. The use of carrangeenan meets the FDA's criteria for GRAS (Generally Regarded as Safe). It is also vegetarian unlike some other thickening and gelling agents.

SHELLAC

Shellac is another place where bugs are the main ingredient for it's production. Shellac is used as a shiny coat on things such as jelly beans, fresh fruits and vegetables, etc. It is used to put a glossy finish on things. It is made from the excretions of Kerria lacca insects that are native to Thailand. Vegetarian lobbyists have repeatedly asked the FDA to require that it be labeled on products that contain shellac as 'coated with insect derived substances. They did not want to go this far, however the FDA, according to Jacobson, did require produce packers to disclose whether any coating used is animal- or vegetable-derived. "But it would be on a placard or on the box of produce, not in bold type on the fruit or vegetable itself," says Jacobson, and not necessarily displayed to grocery shoppers.

GELATIN

Gelatin is used in many packaged foods as a thickening agent. It is used in gummy candy, Jell-O, ice cream and yogurt. According to the USDA, the gelatin that is found in gummy bears and gives them their kid- pleasing texture is created out of several different animal parts, including ligaments, skin, tendons and bones. Though some non-animal versions of gelatin are available, vegetarians are known to avoid packaged foods containing gelatin, unless it's specifically labeled as being derived from a vegetarian source.

BACTERIOPHAGES

Bacteriophages is a food additive that is sprayed on certain foods such as cold cuts and cheeses to prevent viruses from growing on the product. Bacteriophages are a mixture of viruses themselves and they can act to prevent listeria—a microorganism that can be lethal when eaten. "The viruses attack the bacteria and prevent bacterial growth on the food," says Jacobson. "It's actually better than harmless; it's a very clever way to prevent illness."

XANTHAN GUM

Xantan gum is another bacteria--a microbial polysaccharide that's derived from the bacteria Xanthomonas campestris. It is used as a thickening agent. It thickens liquids in very small amounts (concentrations of 0.5 percent or less), therefor, it is generally considered safe for use. It can be found in most bottled salad dressings and it helps to stabilize the dressing, keeping the oil from separating out. What is largely unknown is that Xanthomonas campestris is responsible for the plant disease known as black rot.

"NATURAL" FLAVORS

Natural flavors are the mystery meat of the food-additive world. And while they sound like a good thing—who doesn't want to eat something that's "natural?"—the term can be misleading and confusing. You will find these so-called natural flavors in just about every sort of processed food. They're used to give a "smoked" meat a smoky flavor; give canned peaches back their peachiness; and give an almond-flavored cookie its advertised nuttiness. The mystery is always that when the ingredient isn't specified— and it usually isn't—you don't necessarily know if that "natural flavor" is coming from something you want to eat. For example, you might assume that if canned peaches list "natural flavoring" in the ingredients list, the flavor would be derived from a peach. But according to Jacobson, it could just as likely be referring to apricot extract. Which is harmless, unless perhaps you are allergic to apricots. According to the current Federal Code of Regulations, a natural flavor could be extracted from meat but does not have to specify that if "the function in the food is flavoring rather than nutritional." Once again, it's a case of consumer beware.

The following is a list of possible environmental irritants that you can check for and may be added as a topic. These usually present as some sort of allergy and can be cross checked on the numbers list in the back of the book.

cDUSTS

alfalfa hay
corn grain
cotton gin
dust mites
grain mill
house mixture
mattress
oat rain
prairie hay
Rye grain
Sorghum grain Kafir
soy bean
upholstery
wheat grain
wood

WOODS

alder
birch
cedar
fir
larch
mahogany
maple
monkey pod
oak
pine/white pine
redwood
spruce

PHYSICAL AGENTS

air conditioning
books
burns
car sickness
carbon dioxide
carbon monoxide pois.
carnival rides
change of season
changes is bar. press.

CONT.
PHYSICAL AGENTS

clouds
cold
cold humid air
cold mist
cold mist, serotonin
cold temperatures
computers
cordless, cell hones
dampness
darkness
different colors
different tones
drafts
dryness
electrical sources
electromagnetic fields
exercise
fail

fire alarms
flourescent lights
gas cookstoves
geopathic sources
hairbrush
heat
heating
high altitude
high humidity
hot temperatures
house we live in
humid air
inside air (school/
work)
inside air (home)
loud music
low altitude
low humidity
microwave
mood radiation
moonlight
motion sickness
(sport)
noise sensitivity
outside air
overcast
ozone
physical activity
power lines
radiation
rainwater
seas. affect depression
sea sickness
sirens
smog
spring
summer
swaying motion

television
toothbrush
town we live in
toys
traffic noises
ultraviolet rays
voices in a certain
pitch
washer/dryer
wind
winter
xrays

ELEMENTS

Oxygen
Carbon
Nitrogen
Sulphur

FISH

albacore
anchovy
black bass
channel catfish
codfish
flounder
grouper
haddock
halibut
herring
ling cod
mackeral
mahi-mahi
monkfish
ocean perch

perch
pike
rainbow trout
red snapper
salmon
sardine
shark
sole
steehead trout
sturgeon
swordfish
tunafish
turbot
whitefish

GRAIN & CEREAL

amaranth
barley
barley malt
blue corn
brown rice
buckwheat
corn oat
cornsilk
couscous
farina
gliadin
gluten
kanut
millet
oat
oat bran
popcorn
quinoa
red corn
red wheat

rice
rice bran
rye
teff
wheat bran
wheat germ
white corn
white wheat
white wheat flour
whole wheat
wild rice
yellow corn

NUTS & SEEDS

almond
anise seed
black walnut
brazil nut
caraway seed
cashew nut
chestnut
chia seed
coconut
coriander seed
cumin seed
english walnut
fennel seed
filbert
lax seed
hazelnut
macadamia nut
mustard seed
peanut
pecan
pistachio
poppy seed

psyllium seed
pumpkin seed
sesame seeds
sunflower seed
walnut

CHAPTER 8

Acupressure

What is Acupressure?

Acupressure can also be described as acupuncture without the needles. Acupressure involves the application of manual pressure, typically done with the fingertips) to specific points on the body rather than the use of needles in these same areas as in acupuncture. Traditional Chinese medicine, stands behind the principles that the body has vital energy called "chi" or "qi" which flows through the body along invisible lines of energy flow, called meridians. There are believed to be at least 14 meridians which connect our organs with other parts of our body. Acupuncture and acupressure points lie at various points along those meridians. If this flow of qi, or energy, is blocked at any point on a meridian, it can create certain ailments and lead to disease anywhere along that specific meridian. That is why in certain practices of Acupressure, a practitioner may apply pressure to an acupressure point in the foot to relieve a headache. There is no scientific determination of how acupressure works. However, some theorize that the pressure on the acupressure points may promote the release of natural pain-relieving chemicals in the body, called endorphins. Another theory is that the pressure on the point may somehow effect the autonomic nervous system.

Why do People Try Acupressure?

It is customary that most people will try acupressure as treatment for a specific ailment. Some of the more common ailments are:

*Nausea and vomiting during pregnancy or
   morning sickness
*Motion sickness
*Nausea after surgery
*Nausea due to chemotherapy
*Cancer-related fatigue
*Headache
*Menstrual cramps
*Muscle tension and pain

Although more research is necessary to see the effectiveness of acupressure, studies examining acupressure as treatment for nausea have generally found that it's an effective option. All studies have used a particular point on the inside of the wrist called P6 for nausea. Some of the advantages of acupressure to P6 for nausea are that it

can be self-administered by the patient, and
it is believed to be safe for pregnant women
and those with cancer or other illnesses.

How is Acupressure done?

Acupressure is often administered by an
acupuncturist as the patient lies on a massage table
or other flat surface. Acupressure can also be self-
administered to areas that the patient can reach,
although it is always best to consult a professional
for proper instruction on how to conduct the
procedure. Acupressure is generally done by using
the thumb, finger or knuckle to apply gentle but
firm pressure to a meridian point. The pressure is
often increased for about 30 seconds, held steadily
for 30 seconds to two minutes and then gradually
decreased for 30 seconds. This procedure is often
repeated three to five times on a single point.

The point P6 can be found by turning the arm such
that the palm is facing upwards. You then place
the thumb at the center of the crease of the wrist
(where the hand meets the wrist) and then position
it two finger widths away from the crease towards
the elbow. The point is between the two large
tendons of the arm.

Precautions

Acupressure as a technique should never be painful.
If you are in a situation where you find yourself
experiencing pain, it is important to discontinue
the session. The pressure used should be gentle
over fragile or sensitive areas, such as the face. It
is also of note that individuals with osteoporosis,
recent fracture or injury, people who bruise easily,
have bleeding disorders, circulatory problems
from diabetes, and those using anticoagulant

or antiplatelet medications such as Coumadin (warfarin) that "thin" the blood, should avoid acupressure techniques unless it is conducted under the supervision of a qualified specialist. Acupressure done on pregnant women should be only after they have had a consult with their doctor. Acupressure on the abdominal area or on certain points in the leg during pregnancy are contraindicated. It is also contraindicated to conduct acupressure techniques over open wounds, bruises, varicose veins, or any area that is bruised or swollen.

Side Effects

After an acupressure session, some people may feel soreness at the points where treatment was given. It is also commonly reported that people may feel temporarily lightheaded.

Over the next several pages, you will find an index of the common Acupuncture points that are used in Acupressure. You can check these points and clear them if you find that they are an issue with the patient.

*(361 Regular Points and 20
Extraordinary Points)*

157

Dubi (犊鼻 , St. 35)

Duiduan (兑端 , Du 27)

Dushu (督俞 , U.B. 16)

Ear-Heliao (耳和髎 , S.J. 22)

Erjian (二间 , L.I. 2)

Ermen (耳门 , S.J. 21)

External Xiyan (外膝眼 , See Dubi)

Feishu (肺俞 , U.B. 13)

Feiyang (飞扬 , U.B. 58)

Femur-Futu (股伏兔 , St. 32)

Femur-Juliao (股居髎 , G.B. 29)

Femur-Wuli (股五里 , Liv. 10)

Femur-Zhongdu (股中渎 , G.B. 32)

Fengchi (风池 , G.B. 20)

Fengfu (风府 , Du 16)

Fenglong (丰隆 , St. 40)

Fengmen (风门 , U.B. 12)

Fengshi (风市 , G.B. 31)

Foot-Linqi (足临泣 , G.B. 41)

Foot-Qiaoyin (足窍阴 , G.B. 44)

Foot-Tonggu (足通谷 , U.B. 66)

Foot-Zhongdu (足中都 , Liv. 6)

Fuai (腹哀 , Sp. 16)

Fubai (浮白 , G.B. 10)

Fufen (附分 , U.B. 41)

Fujie (腹结 , Sp. 14)

Fuliu (复溜 , K. 7)

Fushe (府舍 , Sp. 13)

Fuxi (浮郄 , U.B. 38)

Fuyang (跗阳 , U.B. 59)

Gall Bladder (胆囊 , Extra.)

Ganshu (肝俞 , U.B. 18)

Gaohuangshu (膏肓俞 , U.B. 43)

Geguan (膈关 , U.B. 46)

Geshu (膈俞 , U.B. 17)

Gongsun (公孙 , Sp. 4)

Guanchong (关冲 , S.J. 1)

Guangming (光明 , G.B. 37)

Guanmen (关门 , St. 22)

Guanyuan (关元 , Ren 4)

Guanyuanshu (关元俞 , U.B. 26)

Guilai (归来 , St. 29)

Hand-Wangu (手腕骨 , S.I. 4)

Hand-Wuli (手五里 , L.I. 13)

Hand-Zhongzhu (手中渚 , S.J. 3)

Hanyan (颔厌 , G.B. 4)

Head-Linqi (头临泣 , G.B. 15)

Head-Qiaoyin (头窍阴 , G.B. 11)

Head-Wangu (头完骨 , G.B. 12)

Hegu (合谷 , L.I. 4)

Henggu (横骨 , K. 11)

Heyang (合阳 , U.B. 55)

Houding (后顶 , Du 19)

Houxi (后溪 , S.I. 3)

Huagai (华盖 , Ren 20)

Huangmen (肓门 , U.B. 51)

Huangshu (肓俞 , K. 16)

Huantiao (环跳 , G.B. 30)

Huaroumen (滑肉门 , St. 24)

Huatuo Jiaji (华陀夹脊 , Extra.)

Huiyang (会阳 , U.B. 35)

Huiyin (会阴 , Ren 1)

Huizong (会宗 , S.J. 7)

Hunmen (魂门 , U.B. 47)

Jiache (颊车 , St. 6)

Jianjing (肩井 , G.B. 21)

Jianli (建里 , Ren 11)

Jianliao (肩髎 , S.J. 14)

Jianneiling (肩内陵 , See Jianqian)

Jianqian (肩前 , Extra.)

Jianshi (间使 , P. 5)

Jianwaishu (肩外俞 , S.I. 14)

Jianyu (肩髃 , L.I. 15)

Jianzhen (肩贞, S.I. 9)

Jianzhongshu (肩中俞 , S.I. 15)

Jiaosun (角孙 , S.J. 20)

Jiaoxin (交信 , K. 8)

Jiexi (解溪 , St. 41)

Jimai (急脉 , Liv. 12)

Jimen (箕门 , Sp. 11)

Jinggu (京骨 , U.B. 64)

Jingmen (京门 , G.B. 25)

Jingming (睛明 , U.B. 1)

Jingqu (经渠 , Lu. 8)

Jinjin, Yuye (金津，玉液 , Extra.)

Jinmen (金门 , U.B. 63)

Jinsuo (筋缩 , Du 8)

Jiquan (极泉 , H. 1)

Jiuwei (鸠尾 , Ren 15)

Jizhong (脊中 , Du 6)

Juegu (绝骨 , See Xuanzhong)

Jueyinshu (厥阴俞 , U.B. 14)

Jugu (巨骨 , L.I. 16)

Juque (巨阙 , Ren 14)

Kongzui (孔最 , Lu. 6)

Kufang (库房 , St. 14)

Kunlun (昆仑 , U.B. 60)

Lanwei (Appendix 阑尾 , Extra.)

Laogong (劳宫 , P. 8)

Liangmen (梁门 , St. 21)

Liangqiu (梁丘 , St. 34)

Lianquan (廉泉 , Ren 23)

Lidui (厉兑 , St. 45)

Lieque (列缺 , Lu. 7)

Ligou (蠡沟, Liv. 5)

Lingdao (灵道 , H. 4)

Lingtai (灵台 , Du 10)

Lingxu (灵墟 , K. 24)

Lougu (漏谷 , Sp. 7)

Luoque (络却 , U.B. 8)

Luxi (颅息 , S.J. 19)

Meichong (眉冲 , U.B. 3)

Mingmen (命门 , Du 4)

Mouth-Yinjiao (口龈交 , Du 28)

Muchuang (目窗, G.B. 16)

Naohu (脑户 , Du 17)

Naohui (臑会 , S.J. 13)

Naokong (脑空 , G.B. 19)

Naoshu (臑俞 , S.I. 10)

Neck-Futu (颈扶突 , L.I. 18)

Neiguan (内关 , P. 6)

Neiting (内庭 , St. 44)

Nose-Heliao (鼻禾髎 , L.I. 19)

Nose-Juliao (鼻巨髎 , St. 3)

Pangguangshu (膀胱俞 , U.B. 28)

Pianli (偏历 , L.I. 6)

Pishu (脾俞 , U.B. 20)

Pohu (魄户 , U.B. 42)

Pushen (仆参 , U.B. 61)

Qianding (前顶 , Du 21)

Qiangjian (强间 Du 18)

Qiangu (前谷 , S.I. 2)

Qichong (气冲 , St. 30)

Qihai (气海 , Ren 6)

Qihaishu (气海俞 , U.B. 24)

Qihu (气户 , St. 13)

Qimai (瘈脉 , S.J. 18)

Qimen (期门 , Liv. 14)

Qinglengyuan (清冷渊 , S.J. 11)

Qingling (青灵 , H. 2)

Qishe (气舍 , St. 11)

Qiuxu (丘墟 , G.B. 40)

Qixue (气穴 , K. 13)

Quanliao (颧髎 , S.I. 18)

Qubin (曲鬓 , G.B. 7)

Quchai (曲差 , U.B. 4)

Quchi (曲池 , L.I. 11)

Quepen (缺盆 , St. 12)

Qugu (曲骨 , Ren 2)

Ququan (曲泉 , Liv. 8)

Quyuan (曲垣 , S.I. 13)

Quze (曲泽 , P. 3)

Rangu (然谷 , K. 2)

Renying (人迎 , St. 9)

Renzhong (人中 , Du 26)

Riyue (日月 , G.B. 24)

Rugen (乳根 , St. 18)

Ruzhong (乳中 , St. 17)

Sanjian (三间 , L.I. 3)

Sanjiaoshu (三焦俞 , U.B. 22)

Sanyangluo (三阳络 , S.J. 8)

Sanyinjiao (三阴交 , Sp. 6)

Shangguan (上关 , G.B. 3)

Shangjuxu (上巨虚 , St. 37)

Shanglian (上廉 , L.I. 9)

Shangliao (上髎 , U.B. 31)

Shangqiu (商丘 , Sp. 5)

Shangqu (商曲 , K. 17)

Shangwan (上脘 , Ren 13)

Shangxing (上星 , Du 23)

Shangyang (商阳 , L.I. 1)

Shanzhong (膻中 , Ren 17)

Shaochong (少冲 , H. 9)

Shaofu (少府 , H. 8)

Shaohai (少海 , H. 3)

Shaoshang (少商 , Lu. 11)

Shaoze (少泽 , S.I. 1)

Shencang (神藏 , K. 25)

Shendao (神道 , Du 11)

Shenfeng (神封 , K. 23)

Shenmai (申脉 , U.B. 62)

Shenmen (神门 , H. 7)

Shenque (神阙 , Ren 8)

Shenshu (肾俞 , U.B. 23)

Shentang (神堂 , U.B. 44)

Shenting (神庭 , Du 24)

Shenzhu (身柱 , Du 12)

Shidou (食窦 , Sp. 17)

Shiguan (石关 , K. 18)

Shimen (石门 , Ren 5)

Shiqizhui (Seventeenth Vertebra
十七椎 , Extra.)

Shixuan (十宣 , Extra.)

Shousanli (手三里 , L.I. 10)

Shuaigu (率谷 , G.B. 8)

Shufu (俞府 , K. 27)

Shugu (束骨 , U.B. 65)

Shuidao (水道 , St. 28)

Shuifen (水分 , Ren 9)

Shuigou (水沟 , See Renzhong)

Shuiquan (水泉 , K. 5)

Shuitu (水突 , St. 10)

Sibai (四白 , St. 2)

Sidu (四渎 , S.J. 9)

Sifeng (四缝 , Extra.)

Siman (四满 , K. 14)

Sishencong (四神聪 , Extra.)

Sizhukong (丝竹空 , S.J. 23)

Suliao (髎素 , Du 25)

Taibai (太白 , Sp. 3)

Taichong (太冲 , Liv. 3)

Taixi (太溪 , K. 3)

Taiyang (太阳 , Extra.)

Taiyi (太乙 , St. 23)

Taiyuan (太渊 , Lu. 9)

Taodao (陶道 , Du 13)

Tianchi (天池 , P. 1)

Tianchong (天冲 , G.B. 9)

Tianchuang (天窗 , S.I. 16)

Tianding (天鼎 , L.I. 17)

Tianfu (天府 , Lu. 3)

Tianjing (天井 , S.J. 10)

Tianliao (天髎 , S.J. 15)

Tianquan (天泉 , P. 2)

Tianrong (天容 , S.I. 17)

Tianshu (天枢 , St. 25)

Tiantu (天突 , Ren 22)

Tianxi (天溪 , Sp. 18)

Tianyou (天牖 , S.J. 16)

Tianzhu (天柱 , U.B. 10)

Tianzong (天宗 , S.I. 11)

Tiaokou (条口 , St. 38)

Tinggong (听宫 , S.I. 19)

Tinghui (听会 , G.B. 2)

Tongli (通里 , H. 5)

Tongtian (通天 , U.B. 7)

Tongziliao (瞳子髎 , G.B. 1)

Touwei (头维 , St. 8)

Waiguan (外关 , S.J. 5)

Wailing (外陵 , St. 26)

Waiqiu (外丘 , G.B. 36)

Weicang (胃仓 , U.B. 50)

Weidao (维道 , G.B. 28)

Weiguanxiashu (胃管下俞 , Extra.)

Weishu (胃俞 , U.B. 21)

Weiyang (委阳 , U.B. 39)

Weizhong (委中 , U.B. 40)

Wenliu (温溜 , L.I. 7)

Wuchu (五处 , U.B. 5)

Wushu (五枢 , G.B. 27)

Wuyi (屋翳 , St. 15)

Xiabai (侠白 , Lu. 4)

Xiaguan (下关 , St. 7)

Xiajuxu (下巨虚 , St. 39)

Xialian (下廉 , L.I. 8)

Xialiao (下髎 , U.B. 34)

Xiangu (陷谷 , St. 43)

Xiaochangshu (小肠俞 , U.B. 27)

Xiaohai (小海 , S.I. 8)

Xiaoluo (消泺 , S.J. 12)

Xiawan (下脘 , Ren 10)

Xiaxi (侠溪 , G.B. 43)

Xiguan (膝关 , Liv. 7)

Ximen (郄门 , P. 4)

Xingjian (行间 , Liv. 2)

Xinhui (囟会 , Du 22)

Xinshu (心俞 , U.B. 15)

Xiongxiang (胸乡 , Sp. 19)

Xiyan (膝眼 , Extra.)

Xiyangguan (膝阳关 , G.B. 33)

Xuanji (璇玑 , Ren 21)

Xuanli (悬厘 , G.B. 6)

Xuanlu (悬颅 , G.B. 5)

Xuanshu (悬枢 , Du 5)

Xuanzhong (悬钟 , G.B. 39)

Xuehai (血海 , Sp. 10)

Yamen (哑门 , Du 15)

Yangbai (阳白 , G.B. 14)

Yangchi (阳池 , S.J. 4)

Yangfu (阳辅 , G.B. 38)

Yanggang (阳纲 , U.B. 48)

Yanggu (阳谷 , S.I. 5)

Yangjiao (阳交 , G.B. 35)

Yanglao (养老 , S.I. 6)

Yanglingquan (阳陵泉 , G.B. 34)

Yangxi (阳溪 , L.I. 5)

Yaoshu (腰俞 , Du 2)

Yaoyan (腰眼 , Extra.)

Yaoyangguan (腰阳关 , Du 3)

Yemen (液门 , S.J. 2)

Yifeng (翳风 , S.J. 17)

Yinbai (隐白 , Sp. 1)

Yinbao (阴包 , Liv. 9)

Yindu (阴都 , K. 19)

Yingchuang (膺窗 , St. 16)

Yingu (阴谷 , K. 10)

Yingxiang (迎香 , L.I. 20)

Yinlian (阴廉 , Liv. 11)

Yinlingquan (阴陵泉 , Sp. 9)

Yinmen (殷门 , U.B. 37)

Yinshi (阴市 , St. 33)

Yintang (印堂 , Extra.)

Yinxi (阴郄 , H. 6)

Yishe (意舍 , U.B. 49)

Yixi (譩譆 , U.B. 45)

Yongquan (涌泉 , K. 1)

Youmen (幽门 , K. 21)

Yuanye (渊腋 , G.B. 22)

Yuji (鱼际 , Lu. 10)

Yunmen (云门 , Lu. 2)

Yutang (玉堂 , Ren 18)

Yuyao (鱼腰 , Extra.)

Yuzhen (玉枕 , U.B. 9)

Yuzhong (彧中 , K. 26)

Zanzhu (攒竹 , U.B. 2)

Zhangmen (章门 , Liv. 13)

Zhaohai (照海 , K. 6)

Zhejin (辄筋 , G.B. 23)

Zhengying (正营 , G.B. 17)

Zhibian (秩边 , U.B. 54)

Zhigou (支沟 , S.J. 6)

Zhishi (志室 , U.B. 52)

Zhiyang (至阳 , Du 9)

Zhiyin (至阴 , U.B. 67)

Zhizheng (支正 , S.I. 7)

Zhongchong (中冲 , P. 9)

Zhongfeng (中封 , Liv. 4)

Zhongfu (中府 , Lu. 1)

Zhongji (中极 , Ren 3)

Zhongliao (中髎 , U.B. 33)

Zhonglüshu (中膂俞 , U.B. 29)

Zhongquan (中泉 , Extra.)

Zhongshu (中枢 , Du 7)

Zhongting (中庭 , Ren 16)

Zhongwan (中脘 , Ren 12)

Zhouliao (肘髎 , L.I. 12)

Zhourong (周荣 , Sp. 20)

Zhubin (筑宾 , K. 9)

Zusanli (足三里 , St. 36)

162

CHAPTER 9

Affirmations

Patient Affirmations

Affirmations can be a powerful part of healing and clearing blockages in a patient. These affirmations can be repeated in a patients mind while levels are being cleared. Any affirmation can be used depending on the needs of your client. The following are some suggestions to get you started:

I am absolutely certain that:

* I am naturally enlightened.

* My life is blossoming in total perfection.

* I have everything I need to enjoy my here and now. I am the master of my life.

* Everything I need is already within me.
Perfect wisdom is in my heart.

* I am whole and complete in myself.

* I accept all my feelings as part of myself. I
love to love and be loved.

* The more I love myself, the more I have to
give others.

* The more I have, the more I have to give.
The more I give, the more I receive and the
happier I feel.

* I now give and receive love freely.

* I am now attracting loving, satisfying, happy relationships into my life.

* My relationship with is growing happier and
more fulfilling every day.

* I have a perfect, satisfying, well-paying job.

* I love doing my work, and I am richly rewarded, creatively and financially. I am an
open channel of creative energy.

* I am dynamically self-expressive.

* I always communicate clearly and effective-
ly.

* I am now attuned to the divine plan of my
life.

* I now have enough time, energy, wisdom
and money to accomplish all my desires.
* I am always in the right place at the right
time, and successfully engaged in the right
activity.

* It's okay for me to have everything I want!

* This is a rich universe and there's plenty for
all of us. Abundance is my natural state of
being; I accept it now. Infinite riches are now
freely flowing into my life.

* Every day I am growing more financially
prosperous. It's okay for me enjoy myself, and
I do!

* I am relaxed and centered. I have plenty of
time for everything I am now enjoying; I do!

* I feel happy and blissful just being alive.

* I am open to receiving all the blessings of
this abundant universe. I am vibrantly healthy
and radiantly beautiful!

* (You fill in the blank) is coming to me, easily and effortlessly.

* I have a wonderful job with wonderful pay. I
do a wonderful service in a wonderful way.

* The light of God within me is producing
perfect results in every phase of my life now.

* The light with me is creating miracles in my
here and now.

* I give thanks for divine restoration in mind, body, financial affairs, and in my relationships now.

* All things are now working together for good in my life.

* I now recognize, accept and follow the divine plan of my life as it is revealed to me step by step.

* I give thanks now for my life of health, wealth and self-expression. I apply new learning until positive habits are formed.

* Every day, in every way, I'm getting better, better and better. Everything is coming to me easily and effortlessly.

* I am attracting only healthy, positive people in my life. I feel enjoyment in learning.

* I see personal value in learning.

* I am influenced by a person I love and respect. I am involved in the learning process.

* I am interested in the subject and want to learn.

* I can relate new learning to previous experiences. I have the necessary skills to learn.

* What I say next can change the world. I can make a difference in the world.

* I am successful.

* I am surrounded by positive thoughts and emotions. I know what I want.

* I take responsibility for my mistakes and failures and create favorable circumstances from my success.

* I passionately pursue the objects of my desire. I am courageous.

* I apply new learning until positive habits are formed. I acquire knowledge easily.

* Every failure brings forth a seed of success. I cooperate in a spirit of harmony.

* I am nourished by an invisible stream of power. I know how I am.

* I see, feel and believe that I have all that I desire.

* I live in a world of abundance of all my heart desires. I render humble service.

* I transmute my desires into manifestation. I am safe.

* I am persistent.

* I believe in myself.

* I trust and follow my intuition.

* I am responsible for my financial well-being. I take continuous action to achieve my goals.

* I organize knowledge into definite plans of action. I create perfect pictures of my desired results.

* I am honest.

* I live my life with meaning.

* My signatory of averment means my need for safety counts. All my thoughts are equally important.

* I choose how much time I spend with each person. I can learn through...(your choice?)

* I can be healed through touch. I can teach through touch.

* I take responsibility for my own learning (health.) I am –
      a. (name)
      b. (title)

* I am worthy of an abundant income.

* I am worthy of money I earn.

* I have nothing to give or receive but love (shielding, bonding.)

* I do my best. (This is the opposite of "I have to be perfect.")

* I allow people space to grow in their own good time.

* I allow enough time for the learning (healing) process. (The opposite is "I have to suffer

for others; solve the world's problems; intrude on the healing process; etc.)

* I like what I do.

* I attract the people and opportunities that allow me to the work I love.

* I accept all things that may, could or will happen without judgment.

* I open my heart to all things.

* I accept all things that may, could or will happen without criticism.

* I am willing to release all unhealthy cords of attachment.

* I accept all things that may, could or will happen without expectation.

* I open my mind to all things.

* I create what I want.

* I stay grounded while creating what I want.

* I set no limitations.

* I go for what I want; It's my dream.

* Nobody in the world matters right now, only me.

* I focus on the feeling in my body.

* I allow my body to express itself freely.

* The infinite spirit will open the way for
great abundance>

* I am an irresistible magnet for all that be-
longs to me by my divine right.

* I release the pattern in me that created this.

* I am at peace.

* I am worthwhile.

* May our days be touched by luck, brightened
by song and warmed by smiles.

* When we are feeling thankful, life takes on a
deeper richness, a warmer glow.

* Never let the fun go out of your life.

* We have many good things to be thankful
for and many yet to discover.

* Think positive healthy thoughts.

* Spend time with positive, uplifting people
you want to be like.

* Work on your 'people skills' to become more
connected and to enhance limbic bonds.

* Talk to others in loving, helpful ways.

* Surround yourself with great smells.

* Build a library of wonderful experiences.

* Make a difference in the life of someone else.

* This is gonna be a great day.

* God is directing my steps; his favor is surrounding me.

* I am excited about today.

* I expect circumstances to change in my favor.

* I expect people to go out of their way to help me today.

* I expect to be at the right place at the right time.

* I anticipate doors of opportunity to open for me. I expect to have success in my careers.

* I am counting on rising above life's challenges today.

* I am anticipating significance, not mediocrity.

* I refuse to allow my circumstances, my feelings, or my past experiences to dull my experiences for life and imprison me in a negative frame of mind.

* I am committed to living a life that serves a greater purpose.

* We are safe and secure in our world.

* We rise above all limitations.

* New doors will open for truth and peace.

* We need to aspire to increase our vibrational frequency to transcend all limitations.

* I have everything I need to enjoy my here and now.

* I love and appreciate myself just as I am.

Conclusion

I hope that you have enjoyed reading and that you have hopefully been able to open your mind to what an alternative drug free healing journey this technique is. Hopefully using the tools in this book you will be able to get to the point where you can help others with what you have learned. Believe in positive thinking. Negative emotions can hold us back.

Please feel free email me at:

mplescroart@ prodigy.net

You can also visit my website at:

www.marijanelescroartiit.org

Please keep in touch. And feel free to send me others that you know as well.

Happy Healing...

Marijane

The Following pages contain the Numbers and Topic list. This is to be used as a reference when identifying the blockages of your patient...

Numbers List

0 = If you arrive at zero - shift to another level x (times)- For example: The subject of Movement, affected by items 41 (lack of encouragement), 12 (world event), 0 (shift to another level), 3 (self worth), 22 (tribulation), 23 (neurofibulary), 47 (forced), 74 (orthomolecular medicine), 91 (communication), 19 (mold), 66 (epidermis) X = variable that the item is currently stuck at.

THE SYMPTOMS ALL REMAIN UNTIL ALL LEVELS ARE UP TO 1000

A decimal point relates to fine details that are still integrating through the progression of the number previous.

****

1. CORN
  ***Liver (Pectoralis Major Sternal)**
  *Grains, fillers, turn to sugar in the blood

system that in turn effects various organs.
For example: a part of the brain, hypothalamus, stomach, digestive tract, gall bladder,
eyes, high blood pressure, liver, pancreas,
kidney (left), reproductive organs, colon
villa, plaque, makes the body retain weight,
carbohydrates.
*Anti-cancer and anti-viral activity, pos-
sibly induced by corn's content of protease
inhibitors. Has estrogen boosting capabili-
ties. A very common cause of food intolerance linked to the following symptoms:
~Rheumatoid arthritis
~irritable bowel syndrome
~headaches and migraine-related
  epilepsy
~bellyache
~behavior

2. ASSAULT
***Vital (Coracobrachialis Lateral)**
*Issues and events that cause trauma.
Trauma qualifies as any hurt of any kind
that happens to you (physical, emotional,
spiriual, internal or external, past or present.)
*Examples of issues and events:
~A violent attack, either physical or ver-
bal.
*Each assault can compound upon another.
*Each emotion can then make the preceed-
ing assault worsen.
*All our experiences have energetic and
logical reasoning for happening. We can
change and create our own reality from moment to moment.

*Goal intention and understanding the frequency number can heal without drugs. Traumas that effect our future and then change our present and past.

3. WORTH
***Gall Bladder (Anterior Deltoid)**
*The value of something measured by it's qualities or by the esteem in which it is held. A moral or personal value. Merit excellence a field in which a person has proved.
*Worth can affect a majority of life events both positive and negative.
*Self, anything dealing with self; feeling inner peace, balance, internal and external of mental, emotional, and physical.
*ORDER OF LIFE
**Worth may effect the waist, arms, and shoulder. Self concepts retain shoulder pains. Can affect movement and ability to move joints with proper case, comfort with flexibility in all joints.*
*Moving foward in life. Flexibility and fol-low through.
*People's opinion can effect our worth.

4. CHICKEN FAT
*** Lung (Anterior Serratus)**
* Communicaton and assimilation; absorption of fats in the body, the body processsing fat
* Communication in general, thyroid (because communication comes in through the throat), religious beliefs, interference of

feminine output from the body, accumula-
tive fat in areas of the body starting at the
knees and going up just below the navel
(core of the body), communication between
male and female.
* ARCHETYPES
* Communication Malvin's (Malvin is a
neurotransmitter) coating to make contact.
Slow down the current. Chickens have been
violently killed and fat remains affected
which slows the current of communication
between two or more individuals. Chicken
fat relates to communication to Malvin's
neurotransmitter of Neutrons copper with
right and left hemispheres of the brain.
Communication between two objects. People cells corpus collosum, male-female, nation to nation, state to state, etc. Negative-
positive, front-back, top-bottom, side-side,
right-left.
* Combination of many objects, things
worth-communication crosses many meridians. Levels make the communication harder to unscramble, many relationship and behavior can clean up.

5. B-COMPLEX

*Stress, Xiaxi (acupressure point GB43)
*B-complex, base of all nutrients, deals
with the nutrients in everything. Behavior,
the hormones; the spoken and unspoken
word, expression, the tongue, bittersweet
sour taste buds, pancreas-spleen-liver intake and outtake, tongue and heart, intake
thyroid, how life is perceived and how others perceive you; judgment; has to do with

masses and easy way out. – ADDICTIONS
– WORRY STRESS– (Qualifier– hormonal,
food,base of all nutrients), deals with the
nutrition in everything, power, math, vision
(external and external), cingulate system-
ability to shift attention, cognitive flexibility, adaptability, movement from one idea
to another, ability to see options, ability to
go with the flow, ability to cooperate (sym-
toms– OCD, PMS, behavior
*WORRY

6. PERSISTENT
* Central (Anterior Deltoid)
* Something that is consistent, always the
same, not changing, stubborn, opinion and
stuck in one place, no movement.
* CALVES OF LEGS

7. OPINION
* Regulating Yang (Infraspinatus Inferior)
* All opinions, internal and external, relates
to beliefs and judgments–calves, inhibitors.

8. CARL WERNICKE'S AREAS
*Bladder (Peroneus)
* Any trauma to the brain, more analytical
part of the brain.
*CIRCLE OF THOMAS WILLIS
    ~blood clots, veins, spider veins, Neu
rotransmitters, connections, dehydration,
electrolytes, amino acids, mucus

*The lymphatic system; how the body
works with the flow
*THE FLOW OF LIFE-too control-
ling behavior, WORRY, STRESS,
Xiaxi (accupressure point GB43).

9. COPPER
*Tailbone- Coccyx-saccrum
*Plexuses (Crown, Pineal, Throat, Heart,
Diaphragm, Solar, Spleen, Abdominal,
Senital)
* Any increments of money; minerals; completion, connections, right and
left hemispheres, general core connections, top and bottom of money related,
neurotransmitters, electrical current of
body and brain, comprehension, right
and left hemispheres, top and bottom
of body, laterality, centering completion, circuits, electrical charge, gray hair

10. WHY ME
*Triple Warmer (Teres Minor)
* The self, not moving forward, no forward
movement, no change, issues and challenges, hard times, lessons learned, finding the
way to begin.
*Relationship, letting go, allowing enjoy-
ment in/of life, lessons learned
*SECONDARY ELEMENTS

11. HAUNTED
*Kidney (Psoas)
*Will attempt to make forward move-

ment to cause change to visit. Frequently, reoccur, lingering, present in
memory or thought process. Related to past life, can't get rid of.

12.   WORLD EVENTS
***Circulation Sex (Gluteus Medius)**
*Accumulation of energies. World events
can effect timelines and the environment.
Note/music/pitch. An exchange of ideas/
views, opinons, a written state of history
on path of environmental happenings, any
component of energy (accumulation of energies.)
**Effects gait, reflexes, hyoid bone (deals with
balance), cloacal (cavity in which the intestinal,
urinary, and reproductive canals open in human
beings.)*
*This indicates a physical reflex relating to
regeneration, digestion, and elimination,
stepping side to side (related to cross-later-
al) *Ref. Applied Kinesiology Workbook Manual*
*Lymphatic, adrenal stress, cra-
nial stress, hip balance.

13. VIOLENT
***Small Intestine (Quadriceps)**
*Religion- Belief system of perceptions in
need of change; VIOLENT behavior, contact,
expresson.
*Vibration messenger of our transcentdental/
divine nature and highest spiritual aspira-
tions. Uplifting and inspirational. The color
violet's potent vibrations urge transformation, change and purification on all levels of

being.
*Facilitates spiritual growth by accelerating
the release and positive transformation of
old mental/emotional patterns.
*Promotes forgiveness, devotion, service,
loyalty, grace and tenderness. Enhances
meditation, relaxation, contemplation, insight, intuition.
*Symbol of royalty, majesty, power. Helps
dissolve negativity. Exerts a powerful healing influence. Beneficial for all forms of
neurosis. Soothing and tranquilizing for
the nerves. Calms violence and irritability. Beneficial for blood (purification), bone
growth, excess hunger, brain, pineal and
pituitary glands, spleen, kidneys, bladder,
entire system in general.
* Can represent: Intolerance, anger, injustice, restriction, arro-
gance, martyrdom, fanaticism.

14. OLD
* Belt (Palmaris Longus)
*A feeling; dealing with the past; famil-
iarity, ancestry, DNA CODE related, dealing with a past life, old patterns, old beliefs, not willing to let go, relating.

15. SAFE
*Mobility Yang (Supraspinatus)
* Dealing with primary reflexes which deal
with the reptilian brain (survival, bonding, feeling comfortable, being safe, wanting, peace, bonding, COMFORT ZONE.

16.   SKEPTICAL
*Connections, moving forward, hesitant,
fear of unknown, not knowing, misun-
derstand, not integrated, circuits, prefixes,
teeth formation, calcium, bite beliefs, reli-
gion, relating to characteristics, thought

17.   CRUSHED
Stomach Related
*Digestion, worry, grief, or grieveing
*Purposely setting up negative situations to
fail process to move, process to change
*Hurt feelings (physical, emotional, spiritual

18.   RADIAL NERVE
Spleen (Latissimus Dorsi)
*Dealing with the hands; dealing with fine
detail; openness; worth issue; radial nerve
in the elbow
*Has to do with heart and kidneys
*Arm, funny bone, elbow to hand, peo-
ple on your nerves, something that
has to be addressed, self doubt

19.   MOLD
*Old, what is underneath, underlying mo-
tivations; under carpet that no one can see,
smell but cannot see.
*FINGER NAILS- any kind

20. STRONTIUM
*Any kind of mineral, clear substance that holds the bones together, the amino acid (chiclets) (whey); could be higher numbers where things are in space- UNIVERSE
*Similar to copper but more
toxic- Alzheimer's

21. ROSEMARY
*Rosemary can treat headaches, indigestion, nausea, gas and fevers. It is a stimulant and has uses when smoked to help stop smoking (no nicotine) and it helps the lungs with moderate use.
*THE FIVE SENSES; healing herb (that goes along with number 38 = NATURE)

22. TRIBULATION
*Trials, something new; change; moving forward; has to do with alpha, beta, delta, and theta waves
*TRANSFORMATION
*Great misery or distress, as from oppression; deep sorrow
*Also something that causes suffering or distress; affliction; trial

23. NEUROFIBULARY
*Mobility Yin (Rhomboideus Major T3)
*Def: A tiny fiber in the cytoplasm of a neuron which continues on into the nerve processes
*Nerve dealing with another connection

neurotransmitters, nerve that is within the
spinal cord; a disc that branches out to the
central nervous system and could be short
circuited, not allowing integration, causing
discharge and an overflow of energy, connections with people, relationships, other
than self the outer perimeter- to preoccupy
the mind of the exclusion of other thoughts
or feelings, to influence before and against
or in favor of someone or something, preju-
dice bias, to impress favortism in advice
how the body recieives information dealing
with feeling and touch; outward extremi-
ties.
*Sense of being touched by others. An outer
knowing (can be blocked and not recieved).
*Could be short circuited, brain and skin,
outside yourself. Look at the color violet,
use color
*VIOLENT, behavior, con-
tact, expression, valuable

24.   RELIGION
*A belief in how the universe was formed, a
visual concept
*A physical structure taking other con-
ciousness of similar opinions and ideas
*Sulphur 30-cepia, knees-
breasts-eyes, blurry

25.   HELP
*Governing (Trapezius Upper Superior)
*To assist, to aid, to contrib-
ute and to give attention to

26. FIBULAR COLLATERAL LIGAMENT

*Def. Calf bone-one of the longest, thinnest bones in the body. Dealing with the knees, stepping forward in the future, being open minded, joint movement, gelatin, being able to stand up for yourself, holding yourself up, dealing with the tendons and the capillaries, small things that can't be seen, standing up and following through with whatever your idea or concept could be. Amino acids, something is wrong and a correction needs to be made, to cross over, between.

*Collateral Ligament

27. SPITE

*Large Intestines (Tensor Fascia Lata)

*Deliberate, choice, joints in the body, joint and/or joining together

*Plaque- patches of bacteria growth infection in an organic matrix. Scar tissue that form where the layer of myelin covering the nerve fibers is destroyed (by multiple sclerosis). It is a deposit of cholesterol in the arteries possiby causing disease.

*Ligaments, lubrication, 90 degree angles; frequencies, the given and gifted, deliberate; get the job done to perfection, immaturity, no matter what, it's not right, self-punishment, sabotage

28. OVERWHELM

*Deals with fear of routine, deals with the

vision, order, feelings, internal pressure,
veins, chemicals, frontal cortex, being flustered
*Deals with feelings, too
much on your plate.

29. PREOCCUPIED
*Look at what you are doing, not looking at
what the truth is, trying to avoid the truth,
jittery, lack of focus, nervously jumping up
and down, has to do with blood pressure in
general.
*Living something you shouldn't become.

30. OUT OF SORTS
*Usually not in your body, dealing with
the hind brain, basic survival stuff, faulty
connections or shortening connections,
not making proper choices, confused

31. HOPELESSNESS
*Lack of belief, negative thoughts, kynuenic
crenic acid and amino acid dealing with the
ryonia chemical reactions in the brain, connections, pulsating, dealing with the heart.

32. FRUSTRATION

*Dealing with feelings that are unresolved, something that is not accomplished, feeling of discontentment, confused or encumbered; lack of power, dealing with the eyes, and how you see it.

*High and low blood pressure in the moment, lack of or too much salt or sodium, circulation.

*Hysteria, energy imbalance, panic attacks, lifestyle imbalance.

33. MIND BOGGLING

*Cannot figure it out logically, order, organization, related to the right hemisphere of the brain (gestalt), iron being the key function of the brain, iron deficiency can weaken your attention, memory and learning ability.

*Dealing with synthesis integration and formation, deformities or deformation, the big picture, faces, memory of faces, wrinkles on the face, joint inuries and jet lag.

34. WORRY

*Stomach (Pectoralis Major Clavicular)

*Issues of the stomach, digestion, premenstrual syndrome, hormones, butterflies in the stomach, fidgety, nervous disorders of the stomach, feeling anxiety

35. HYSTERICAL

*Dehydration or hydration, mineral imbalance, fluids in or on the brain. Minerals affecting the brain, the gray matter, eyes, blurred vision, signals of the brain not getting to the eyes, expression, focus of vision or focal point, inner strength, environmental sensitivity

36. INTIMIDATION

*Regulating Yin (Pectoralis Minor Sup)
*Bad news, anything dealing with society, challenging your beliefs of feelings, intake
*Repetitive strain injury, lymphatic system, carpal tunnel syndrome, movement of the neck, shoulder and arms, upper body movement, incontinence, potassium, bladdeer, the teeth, happiness, joy of life, keytones, pressure in general (inner and outer)

37. HURT

*Like crushed but not as severe
*Has to do with the heart and circulation; also yang; the hips and any fat accumulation around the bottom of the hip area, the head of the femur and how it fits in the pelvic bone, judgement, loss of power, not giving up but giving into others

38. RESCUE
*The inability to follow through with some-
thing; unseen blocks, error, bile ducts and
pancreas, inside of the vein or artery, pushing the blood throught the vein, lymph's
rejuvenation relieved, comfortable, bliss
*Turine, Strontium, Acetylcholine

39. ISOLATION
*Feeling of being alone, could be house
bound, no social outlet, creating a prison
atmosphere, aloneness, victim
*CONCIOUSNESS, no conception of aware-
ness, a knowing of a situation without control to change it, creating mazes, isolating
circumstances that are out of order and ar
not being linked together.

40. VAGUS NERVE
*Legs, standing up for self, brain
to toes, being centered, good foundation, grounded, focused.

41. LACK OF ENCOURAGEMENT
*Insecure, pointing at the oth-
er person, environment.

42. LACK OF OPPORTUNITIES
*Hysterical, panic attack, feeling of
loss, choice and choosing correctly,
in another path, life style change.

43. OSCILLATION
*Back and forth, indecisive, unable to make
decisions, unwilling to change, lack of
trust, hidden meaning, joint injuries, ankles, knees, wrists and elbows, something
that you do not want to face, wrinkles

44. OPPRESSED
*Made to feel bad by others,
*Smudge: Burn green candle in water until
it goes out, burn bundle of sage leaves, wild
sage
*Feeling of excess weight on the emo-
tions, dealing with authority.

45. DEPRIVED
*Feeling sorry for one's self, denial, whiny,
scaring, excess of thickening, skin callous,
emotionally growing a second outer layer of
skin
*Small intestines
*Bruising easily on the forearm, thighs and

calves that turn purple/blue
*BIOFLAVANOID

46. ANALYTICAL
*In your head, thinking too much, getting
in a rut and not shifting, conscious control,
stagnant, holding the breath
*Ileum

47. FORCED:
Stomach (Pectoralis Major Clavicular)
*Strained and also sprained, ankles, ribs
*Adrenals
*Pulls off your balance and making you
overcomplensate, problems making choices.

48. FURIOUS
Regulating Yin (Pectoralis Minor Sup)
*Not seeing anything but negative emo-
tion, rage, being reactive instead of proactive, self-punishment, not able to col-
laborate in any relationship, unable to
think how other people feel, care issue, deep seated, don't know why

49. HYPOCRITICAL
*Doing something you should not do, doing
something that really is not the truth, getting sidetracked, out of now, in the future,
in the past-states of
*Possible other dimensions

50. RITUAL
*Religious, spiritual, routine, positive
habits, a system of rites, act or action.

51. HEART
*Heart (Subscapularis)
*Actual physical organ, dealing with the
feelings, the elbows, circulation, sorry,
anger/happiness, the gallbladder, feeling of being secure, abnormal heart
beats, bringing the body to center.

52. HOMESICK
*Anything relating to the past, the home,
family, roots, feelings, the skeletal system,
dryness and cracking of bones, osteoporosis, feeling of being left out of a situation.

53. LETHARGIC
*Tired, sleepy, depressed, with-
drawn, living like a hermit, pineal gland, darkness and light,
blood flow, the toes, fine detail.

54. LUSTING
***Triple warmer (Teres Minor)**
***Circulation sex (Gluteus Maximus)**
*Happy, sexual, lusting for the future,
something that you cannot get
*Pus, pores, boils

55. OPPOSING
*Resisting, catatonic, repetitive, self-absor-
ved, unwilling
*Uncooperative, temper tantrums,
white cells, brain related, survival, paralysis of the brain, over exag-
gerated, balance, to anticipate.

56. JITTERY
*Feeling shaky, obsessing, decision making,
somewhat off balance, terrified
*Thyroid, hormones related.

57. HOLDING BACK
*Unwillingness to let go of the old, con-
stipation, swelling of membranes, going along with the crowd but really wanting to do it, terror

58. GRIEF
*Deep sorrow, deep physical, left elbow,
receiving and pursuit, swelling, weeping,
lethargic, general scar tissue
*The heart, aorta, rhythm of the heart, an-
eurysm in the aorta, dealing with the back
chamber of the heart, lack of opening of the
heart
*Black (from color awareness guide). A
powerful and often misunderstood color.
Black represents the dark and comforting
womb of the Mother, deep silence, the void.
*The dark and fertile soil which supports
our gestation/learning processes until, lilke
the sprouting seed, we emerge into the light
of our inner wisdom, personal power and
self-mastery. Symbol of the 'dark side' of
human nature, all that is unknown, mysterious and hidden from the conscious mind.
*Historically, black has been associated
with meance, evil and negativity. Black is
none of these; it has simply become an external projection, a 'scapegoat' for our fear
of our own 'dark side', our fear of the unknown. Represents the introspective personal journey into the depths of being' it is
not a journey of fear.
*Black is considered formal, an image of

dignity and power. Stabilizing and ground-
ing. Offers a sense of security and self-
containment.
*Restricts and confines one's emotions as-
sisting introspection, contemplation and
inner stillness.
*Signifies secrecy, sorrow, mourn-
ing, loss, death. Can present: rage,
fear, doubt, denial, superstition, misunderstanding, grief, guilt, lack.

59. HESITANT

*Holding back, unwillingness to make small
changes
*Proper place, proper time, protein absorp-
tion in all of the glands, glutamine precur-
sor to GABA, depression, high anxiety, high
blood pressure, feeling of a subtle push.

60. JEALOUSY

*Virus, polio, DNA code, a thickness similar
to mucus that coats the DNA code, toxins,
stiffness in the body, transformation, having to do with the five elements, change,
can be aware or unaware, patterns–cycle,
circumference, equilibrium.

61. SATISFIED
   *The area underneath the tongue, the
   tongue and the tase buds, uvula at the
   end of the soft pallet, saliva, pressure in
   the ears, the nodes on the ear, villa in
   the ear, vibration of sounds in the head,
   nerves, overabundance, cranial lock.

62. WATER (H20)
   *Hydrogen bonding in water, rain, hot and
   cold, internal and external, vertical, lying
   flat, values, lying, not telling the truth
   *Knees, pelvic bones, ball of the foot,
   parathyroid glands, purivicy

63. ABUSE
   *Frontal cortex, bones in the fingers on the
   left hand, internal, radical, surgery, in want
   of attention, imbalance, regret, change,
   perception, dissolution, cingulate (OCD
   behaviors in the brain or negative behavior
   patterns)
   *Obsessive to the point of self-sabotage,
   under mind.
   *Attitude behavior damaging one's self to
   creating self or other instead of letting enjoyment of life prevail.
   *Being narrow minded, having the rash on
   the upper arm, self-inflicted challenged
   image, conscientiousness
   *Stature, posture, and pose of

an individual domineer.

64. EXPECTATIONS
*The unusable, dealing with the out-
side perimeter of the universe, taking one path in life then it changing,
goals, achieve, motivation, sleeping patterns, protein, an actualization of deep
understanding, praise of oneself.

65. REGROUP
*The waste around the physical waist,
flow of the blood in the valves in the
body, open portions, shuffled.

66. EPIDERMIS
*Skin, anything on the outside of the body,
encumbrances coming to the surface, in
seven layers, hiding something for protec-
tion.
*Vitamin C

67. NAUSEA
*From Niacin, non production of bile, no

digestion, not in the body, amino acids, enzymes.
*The liver, gallbladder, spleen, pancreas.

68. HALOPERIDOL (HALDOL)
*A drug used when an alcoholic is in DT's
(detox), Vitamin C, arteries, the flow of
blood, the flow of life, tense, irritable, inner pressure, low self-esteem, scurvy, scar-
city (short supply), cracking of epidermal
layer of the lips and the orifices, herpes.

69. HEADACHES
*Not enough light, chakras, not enough
sunshine, Vitamin D, the way the light
reflects into the body through the eyes
and cranials, function pineal gland,
the position of the nose in the internal cranial bones, bacteria, elemen-
tal functoning of an underlying cause,
static electricity, seizures, cranial.

70. OVALBUMIN
*Egg white, eggs, protein, sexuality, com-
munication, also dealing with subject number 7 opinion, Melvin, Avidin, neurotransmitters, male/female communication, libido,
DHEA, ego, kidneys, hormones and hor-

mones in the glands, gelatin, hypothalamus

71. OXALIC ACID
*Causing underlying deficiency of oils and
fats in the body, the heart being the indi-
cator of the thought process, blocks ab-
sorptiion of proteins, constant turmoil,
never seeming to work, no focus, no movement, corpuscles, plaque, kidney stones,
belligerent, cellulite in the thighs, body
clock, assimilation of senses, fluid part of
the body and taste, chakras and meridians, color emotions, climate/spring, summer, fall and winter, no connection to
make things work, constant disruption.

72. HEART ARTERIES
*Feelings, oppressed feel-
ings, hypersensitive, hyperten-
sion, clogged arteries, sea salt.

73. FIBROIDS (FIBROMYOMA)
*Def: A benign tumor that contains a large
amount of fibrous tissue.
*Uterine, fibroids are like tumors,
past life issues and challenges, estrogen imbalance, iron deficiency, blad-

der problems, past life programs, large
fibroids may exert pressure on the bladder causing problems with the bladder
and also causing bowel incontinence.

74. ORTHOMOLECULAR MEDICINE
*Holistic healing, herbs

75. HAND ACCUPRESSURE
*Tactile, tools, deals with the hands, ac-
cupressure points, pulse, meridian.

76. HOLMIUM (HOLH-ME-EM)
*A metallic element of the minerals rare to
the earth. It is a toxic metal.
*The following are possible effects from
contact with this metal: polarity, homolateral, inner ear, numbness in the tips of
the fingers, nail bed, distressed nerves,
hyperactivity, mucus, hypersensitivity, too
alkaline, unable to keep a balance of alka-
line/acid in the organs, enzymes, imbalance of amino acids, the retina and how
color enters the body, failure and failing to
succeed. Group that occurs with yttrium
and forms highly magnetic compounds
are literally soft, malleable in gravity.

77. HABITUAL
*Always with a topic, old patterns,
fear, cold feet, apprehension, dis-
may, dread, fright, horror, panic.

78. NAVIGATING IN WATER
*Breast cancer, boating, swimming, whin-
ing, puberty, juvenile diabetes, hemo-
philiac, blood clotting, scaring, ruptured
appendix, search for a meaning in life.

79. FACET ASPECT OF THE FACE
*Never knowing the truth, wrinkles, dark
circles under the eyes, paralysis, how we
look at life and how life looks back at us,
social aspects, memory, contingencies.

80. VISION
*Actual physical vision, how we look
at things, how we perceive, colors, intensities, focus, crispness.

81. RAIN
*Weather, rain, tornadoes, windstorms,

solid, liquid, gases, hydrogen, calm before
the storm, temperature changes, purivicy,
lymph glands (under the arms), circulation,
breast cancer, sinuses, micro organisms,
gray matter in the brain
*Climate/environment, latitude, longitude,
grids.
*Reflexes.

82. OBSTRUCTIONIST
*Self-sabotage, stuck in repeated pat-
ters, obsessive compulsive, cingulet brain,
extreme frustration, person could have a
photographic memory for shapes, spine
is inverted, slight physical build, metabolism is shut down, gifted people.

83. YEARNING
*Calcium deficiency, skeletal issues,
weak bones, problems with the pelvic area, sequencing, present life issues, living in the future, sexual re-
jection, expression of the soul.

84. PIG OUT
*To binge, too much, can accelerate aging,
clogged pores and glands, swelling, being
overly repetitious, or redundant, overdoing,

olfactory gland (sense of smell), fungus.

85. QUAGMIRE
*Stuck in a pattern, something you can't get out of, patterning, choices, pulsating, consistent negative energy, nerves, electromagnetic fields.

86. TENDS TO EXPECT THE WORST
*Gloomy, temporary low red blood cell count, low iron, liver dysfunction, liver flukes
*The shoulders, posture, rotator cuff (usually the right side)
*Receiving, vitamin absorption.
*To take blame, admit.
*Spine- Thoracic level 4, Thyroid.

87. DECEMBER 2nd
*Past life tragedy, not moving forward, separaton from a loved one, some kind of order, low vibration energy
*Time lines, time cells, dates
*Post traumatic stress

88. MEMORY OF FACES
*Details, memory, sounds, tones, vestibular system (hearing), bones in the face

89. WEAKNESS
*Lacking, fail, capacity, resistance, irresistible desire, structure, physical, emotional, mental, pelvic floor foundation, coolness, shades of emotional imperfection.

90. SALIVA
*Anger (like spitting), mucous membranes, breath, parasites, mucous, lungs, bronchial lobes, vaginal, semen, asthma.

91. COMMUNICATION
*Ritual of spoken word, body language, movement, articulation, circuits of energy of understanding, act of sounds, voice, experience, gestures, tone, speech inflections, meanings of intention, contact, relationships, attunement, co-creation
*Expiration of sound through intimidation, end experimentation with increased ability at total discrimination.
*Ability to categorize objects according to sound clues with vocabulary, hair

follicles, the throat, vocal cords, lips.

92. FEELINGS
*Unjustified, thoracic, lymphatic sys-
tem, touch, epidermis issues, in the body
and outside of the body, how the world is
processed, circulation, effecting actions,
thoughts, organs, beliefs, moods, behavior.
*How we look at life as a whole, move-
ment, motivation, situations and issues, positive and negative.

93. JUDGEMENT
*Judgement of others or ourselves, making
a change or a shift, fungus, lower extremi-
ties, coagulation of the blood, immune system breaking down, mold, enzymes, Epstein
bar syndrome, dormant ringworm in the
lower bladder, color definition
*Vitamin K

94. KYNURENIC UREMIC ACID
*Hemolytic uremic syndrome, molitho-
lites acid, malonylurca acid, hyaluronic acid
(amino acid non-essential)- a mucopoly-
saccharide found in the ground substance
of connective tissue which acts as a binding

protective agent. Also found in the synovial
fluid, vitreous and aqaeous humors in the
eye, fuction of the body blood lymp, cata-
racts, feeling behaviors, brain parts, deep
limbic system, moods, irritabilty, increases
negative thinking, perceptions of events.
*Perception, how we perceive the world
around us, hearing, vision, touch.
*Tastebuds, taste receptors, smell receptors,
tastants.
*Decreases motivation, flood of emo-
tions, inhibits sleep problems, increases or decreases sexual respon-
siveness, social isoloation.

95. XLIUM

*Minerals, physical, tactile, metals, feel-
ings, chitlins, red blood cells, immuno-
globulin level (gluten sensitivity), lacteal
system, pulse of the glands (23) and eyes
at (14), unresolved emotional issues, due to
resentment and embarassment, the rotator
cuff in the shoulder (usually left side), issues with the mother, belief system, being
ornery and persecuted, polarity beliefs.

96. SECURITY

*Small intestinal issues, swelling, vomiting
*Anus sphincter muscle, imbalance, geo-
desic, shapes, pyramid, ayurvedic medicine, the four elements, actual pulse

of the body accelerated, beliefs-before
you ask questions of another person.

97. KETONES

*Sweetness of life
*Contain the carbonyl group (c=o) bonded
to two atoms of carbon instead of one carbon and one hydrogen as in aldehydes.
They are liquids or low melting point sol-
ids, slightly soluble in water, often having a sweet smell. An example is propane
acetone, CH3, COCH3o, Which is used as a
solvent.
*Organs, pancreas, not enjoying life, not
as happy as should be, the outer layer
of the skin, the seventh layer, translu-
cent, the left corner of the eye, the finger nail matrix has pinkish color, chemical imbalance, under layer of a scab the
mucous, upper pallet in the mouth.

98. WANTING

*Waiting-31, 38 up on pinky, diagnostics,
just right before the beginning, salt, hydration, pollens, timing, depression, eye disease with cone shapes.

99. RISKY

*Similar to jittery, a big step, pigment cells of the retina, hanging out, not moving forward, sour taste, very tip of the tongue, dust, extreme sensitivity to warmer temperatures, equator, exposure to exhaust fumes.

100. RECOVERY

*Recovery details = 15, 91, 51, 21, 59
*Circumference, dealing with circles, routine, lesions, qualifications, shifts, pollens, palate, placebo, bioflavonoid, sense of taste, brain plasticity
*An act, instance, process, or duration of recovery. A return to a normal condition.
*Something gained or restored in recovery. The obtaining of usable substance from unusable source, such as waste material, the final verdict or judgement in a case.

101. REPETITION

*Repeating old patterns, renewal, mazes, looks like it is but is not, fung shui, deck of cards

102. RIDICULOUS
*Clues, mediator, soft pallet, rhythm, mela-
nin, pigment, racism
*SOMETHING SO OBVIOUS

103. RESENTMENT
*Suffixes
*bitter indignation or unfair treatment

104. DAUNTED
*Make someone feel intimidated, appre-
hensive, discourage, deter, demoralize, put
off, dishearten, vanquish, be afraid of fear,
doubt, control, restrain
*Worth issue, to feel slightly frightened or
worried about their ability to achieve.
*Transcutaneous electrical nerve stimu-
lation: A form of electrical anesthe-
sia used to block pain perception.

105. PROCESSING MONEY
*Being successful with earning money
*Elements with copper and nickel
*Negotiate/negotiable in context with
financial security. Always in fear
of lack, never having enough.

106. RAILROADS, TRANSPORTATION
*Vehicles to move forward with assistance.

107. ALCOHOLISM
*Sugar, processing of sugar in the body,
candida albacons ('why me' & opinion) to
raise to 137 to shift.
*Alcoholism = 53, 23, 43, 22, 13, 7

108. DYSLEXIA
*Def: Developmental reading disorder
(DRD) is not caused by vision problems but
rather with the brain's ability to recognize
and process symbols. Children with DRD
may have trouble rhyming and separating
the sounds in spoken words. These abilities
appear to be critical in the process of learning to read and spell.
*Low calcium, suicidal, gross
thoughts, minerals, bulimia, numbness, MS, lack of enthusiasm, most
likely to succeed, self sabotage, some-
where a positive side of things.

109. PROPER PLACEMENT
*Sequencing, inspiration, possibilities

110. HAUNTED/WHY ME

111. VINDICTIVE

113. SINISTER
*Giving the impression that some-
thing harmful or evil is happening or will happen. Ex)
there was something sinister
about that murmuring voice.

114. OLD AND REPEATING PATTERNS

115. REJOICE
*Glee, happy, contentment

116. ANDRODEATERIFTY
*Corn/Skeptical/Haunted
*MS-Multiple Sclerosis, MS
*Adrnoturo, Dystrophy/Heal

*Dystrophy is any condition of abnormal development, usually due to malnutrition, especially denoting the degeneration of muscles.
*HPV (Human papilloma virus), Beta Hemolytic Strep group B, Secretin, Staphylococcus Aureus, Rett Syndrome, Tay-Sachs, Formaldehyde, Obesity, hyperplastic, gynecoid, hypertrophic, size, number of fat cells.

117. DECEPTION
*Multiple Sclerosis-extent and site of myelin (that encircles the nerves) destruction.
*Parkinsons (shaking palsy)-causes include decreased dopamine levels.
*The act of convincing another to believe information that is not true, or not the whole truth as in certain types of half truths.

119. RESCUE
*Recovery, mold
*Autoimmune system, Auditory

121. YIELD
*Triangle, yellow, hula hoops,

shades, inerements, healing, 1
use yield to mean quality.

124. EXPERIENCES

125. DIABETES
*(Corn + Help) Indicates Diabetes, sweet-
ness of life, and blood sugar in blood
stream. Raise to 133 to shift.
*Diabetes- 7, 23, 2, 11, 97, 1, 67

133. CORN/MIND BOGGLING

137. `CORN/HURT

140. (CORN + VAGUS NERVE)
*Deals with cancer. RAisse to 160 to shift.
*Core of cancer is 20%, Polio 16%, Paraton-
silar 8%
*Parasites 40%, Mold 17%, Nutritional 54%

*Overlap of Simian 40% of all of these.
*Cancer-79, 70, 11, 7, 33

150. MONEY
*Commodities such as gold or silver is legally established as an exchangeable equivalent of other commodities and used as a measure of their comparative values on the market.
*The official currency, coins and negotiable paper notes are issued by a government. Beliefs about money, money issues, unable to balance financial statement, always in fear of lack of money and resources, never having enough, religious beliefs, money, and different classes of people.

151. RADIANT
*To shine within

153. LETHARGIC/CORN/COARSE
*Has to do with the pinky finger, hesitation, numerology, small intestines, brain, lesions on the brain, buoyancy, never working out the way you wanted it to, self hate, self inflicted, knowing the patterns of behavior.

168. VITAMIN C: BIOFLAVANOIDS

202: TEMPLATE, PATTERNS

215. ASSAULT/SAFETY

313. HOPELESSNESS AND VIOLENT

333. SELVES
*Schizophrenia related
*Rapid succession of incomplete and un-
connected ideas.
*Hallucinations/illusions-false sensory per-
ceptions with no basis in reality.
*Withdrawl-disinterest in ob-
jects, people, or surroundings.

512. HEART/WORLD EVENT/
NO WAY OUT

546. ULTIMATE RESISTING ENERGY

555. ROUGH TERRAIN

901. INSTANTANEOUS

903. COPPER/WORTH

905. EVIDENCE

**907. PINKY THOUGHT PRO-
CESS BODY BRAIN**

ADDENDUM:

The following are some other topics that may be found while working on a patient. They may coincide with other topics and other numbers, so be sure to always cross reference this list.

Abundance = 9, 12, 15. 51, 75,83
Abuse = 8, 6, 32
Actions-follow through = 11, 45, 75
Alcoholism = 53, 23, 43, 22, 13, 7
Attracting money = 4, 37, 47, 73
Auric holes = 3, 9, 14
Bliss = 2, 12, 15, 21, 25, 51, 79, 97, 98
Cancer = 7, 11, 33, 79
Diabetes = 1, 2, 7, 11, 23, 67, 97
Injury = 19, 24, 29, 48
Learning Letters Manifestations = 8, 11, 19, 38, 47, 67, 83, 96
Light = 3, 48, 55, 57, 75, 98
Light-Sound = 8, 18, 19, 41
Lose weight = 8, 37, 46, 51, 74
Love = 8, 12, 14, 21, 28, 42, 65, 66
Miracle = 10, 34, 65, 68, 75
Movement = 0, 3, 12, 19, 22, 23, 47, 66, 74, 91
Money = 105, 150
Neurological = 11, 22, 33, 44, 55, 66, 77, 88, 99
Order = 5, 45, 48, 75, 76
Fraction = 16, 50, 55, 99, 101
Opposite = 18, 36, 43, 71, 94
Mirror Image = If numbers are found that have their mirror image (Ie. 21 and 12, 34, and 43, etc) then this may be a topic of consideration.
Organization = 33, 69, 73, 100

Peace = 7, 9, 23, 33, 81, 89
Power = 42, 62, 67
Problem = 6, 16, 26, 36, 86, 96
Prosperity = 5, 15, 40, 51, 96, 94
Hostaglandin (Accupressure point) E-2 =
Cause of Allergy= 3, 8, 10, 38
Reading Comprehension = 8, 52
Recovery = 15, 21, 51, 59, 91
Seizure = 26, 34, 43, 62
Smitten = 35, 47, 49, 61, 65, 67, 84
Spontaneous– Reality and Timing = 15, 38, 39, 92, 98
Scar Repair = 11, 21, 23, 36, 41, 43, 68
Swelling = 2, 7, 12, 16
Surgical = 2, 12, 41, 87
Trust = 6, 8, 47, 53
Vindictive = 1, 2, 8, 9, 11

For numbers that are not in the list, use the multiplication table on the next page, or you can find a larger version which can be downloaded on the website at:

www.marijanelescroartiit.org

MULTIPLICATION CHART (Up to 15 times table)

Here is a multiplication chart that will help you to revise your times tables from the 1 times table up to the 15 times table.

X	1	2	3	4	5	6	7	8	9	10	11	12	13	14	15
1	1	2	3	4	5	6	7	8	9	10	11	12	13	14	15
2	2	4	6	8	10	12	14	16	18	20	22	24	26	28	30
3	3	6	9	12	15	18	21	24	27	30	33	36	39	42	45
4	4	8	12	16	20	24	28	32	36	40	44	48	52	56	60
5	5	10	15	20	25	30	35	40	45	50	55	60	65	70	75
6	6	12	18	24	30	36	42	48	54	60	66	72	78	84	90
7	7	14	21	28	35	42	49	56	63	70	77	84	91	98	105
8	8	16	24	32	40	48	56	64	72	80	88	96	104	112	120
9	9	18	27	36	45	54	63	72	81	90	99	108	117	126	135
10	10	20	30	40	50	60	70	80	90	100	110	120	130	140	150
11	11	22	33	44	55	66	77	88	99	110	121	132	143	154	165
12	12	24	36	48	60	72	84	96	108	120	132	144	156	168	180
13	13	26	39	52	65	78	91	104	117	130	143	156	169	182	195
14	14	28	42	56	70	84	98	112	126	140	154	168	182	196	210
15	15	30	45	60	75	90	105	120	135	150	165	180	195	210	225

Bibliography

1. "Acids" (2021, July 24th) In Wikipedia. https://en.wikipedia.org/wiki/Acid
2. "Applied kinesiology" (2021, May 14th) In Wikipedia. https://en.wikipedia.org/wiki/Applied_kinesiology
3. Beijing College of Traditional Chinese Medicine, Essentials of Chinese Acupuncture, Foreign Languages Press, 1980
4. William H. Bates, M.D., The Bates Method for Better Eyesight Without Glasses, Holt Paperbacks, 1971
5. Tom and Carole Valentine with Douglas P. Hetrick, D.C, Applied Kinesiology, Muscle Response in Diagnosis, Therapy & Preventive Medicine, Healing Arts Press, 1987
6. Michael Reed Gach. PH.D. And Beth Ann Henning, Dipl.,A. B. T. Acupuncture for Emotional Healing, Bantam Books, 2004
7. Paul E. Dennison and Gail E. Dennison, Educational Kinesiology In- depth, Revised 1995, Edu-Kinesthetics, Inc., 1984
8. Gail E. Dennison and Paul E. Dennison, The Visioncircles Handbook. Edu-Kineshetics, Inc., 1993
9. Paul E. Dennison and Gail E. Dennison. Brain Gym Handbook. Edu- Kinesthetics, Inc., 1986
10. Paul E. Dennison, Ph. D and Gail E. Dennison, Edu-K for Kids, Edu-Kinesthetics, Inc, 1984
11. Don Lepore, The Ultimate Healing System, Course Manual. Woodland Books, 1988

12. Dr. Susan Walker, Retained Neonatal Re-

flexes: A Patient's Companion, San Berdino Ca, 2013

13. David M. Oshinsky, Polio An American Story, The Crusade That Mobilized the Nation Against the 20th Century's Most Feared Disease, Oxford University Press, 2005

14. Mark L. Batshaw, M.D., editor, Children with Disabilities, Fourth Edition, Paul H. Brooks Publishing Co, 1997

15. Paul E. Dennison and Gail E. Dennison, Brain Gym Handbook, The Student Guide to Brain Gym, Second Edition, Edu-Kinesthetics, Inc., 1997

16. F. Batmanghelidj, M.D., Your Body's Many Cries For Water, Second Edition, Global Health Solutions, Inc., 1997

17. Judith Bluestone, The HANDLE Institute, 2001

18. John E. Upledger and JON D. Vredevoogd, Craniosacral Therapy, Eastland Press, 1983

19. James D. Watson and Andrew Barry, DNA, Alfred A. Knopf, 2003

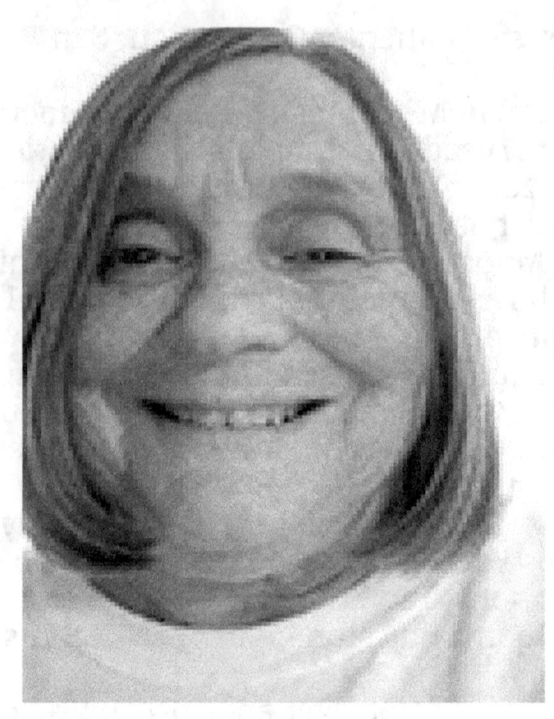

ABOUT THE AUTHOR

Marijane Lescroart has been a holistic
practitioner of her technique for approximately
30 years. She discovered her technique through
years of research and study in an effort to
help her own son's condition with severe food
allergies. Through the years she has compiled
a wealth of knowledge through techniques such
as Brain Gym, Applied Kinesiology, Acupuncture
and other holistic approaches. She has a
Masters in Brain Gym 101, Vision Circles and
Brain Gym In depth therapy. She continues
today to help patients to clear their blockages
and has a passion for helping them to heal
naturally without medications. When Marijane
is not hard at work in her practice, she can be
found spending time with her 4 children in
Santa Rosa, California where she has lived since
1985.

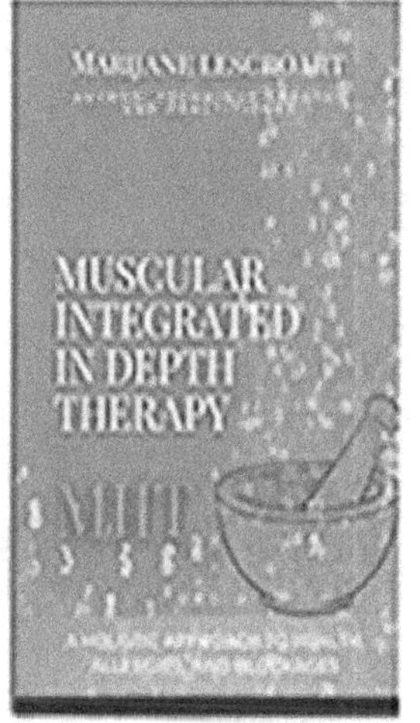

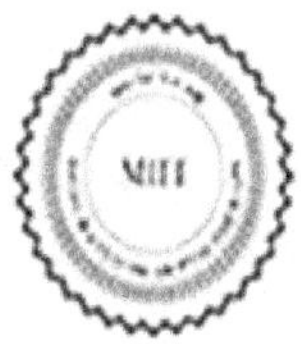

THANK YOU FOR READING!!
FOR FREE PATIENT WORKSHEET
DOWNLOADS AND MORE INFORMATION VISIT

WWW.MARIJANELESCROARTIIT.ORG

www.ingramcontent.com/pod-product-compliance
Lightning Source LLC
Chambersburg PA
CBHW070825250726
48662CB00003B/1085